The History of American Homeopathy

The History of American Homeopathy

From Rational Medicine to Holistic Health Care

John S. Haller Jr.

Rutgers University Press
New Brunswick, New Jersey, and London

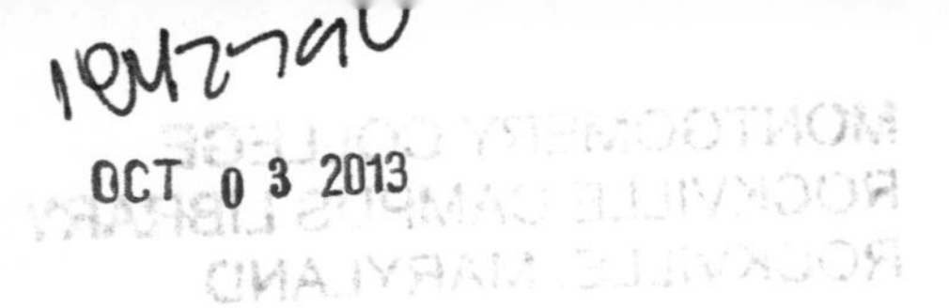

First paperback printing, 2013

Library of Congress Cataloging-in-Publication Data

Haller, John S.
The history of American homeopathy : from rational medicine to holistic health care / John S. Haller Jr.
p. ; cm.
Continues: The history of American homeopathy : the academic years, 1820–1935 / John S. Haller Jr. c2005.
Includes bibliographical references.
ISBN 978-0-8135-6158-5 (pbk : alk. paper)
ISBN 978-0-8135-4583-7 (hard : alk. paper)
1. Homeopathy—United States—History—19th century. 2. Homeopathy—United States—History—20th century. I. Title.
[DNLM: 1. Homeopathy—history—United States. 2. History, 19th Century—United States. 3. History, 20th Century—United States. 4. Homeopathy—trends—United States. WB 930 H185ha 2009]

RX51.H33 2009
615.5'32—dc22

2007048025

A British Cataloging-in-Publication record for this book is available from the British Library.

Visit our Web site: http://rutgerspress.rutgers.edu

Manufactured in the United States of America

For
Peter and Jon

Do I contradict myself?
Very well then I contradict myself,
(I am large, I contain multitudes.)

Walt Whitman,
"Song of Myself"

CONTENTS

Foreword

In 1978 Dr. Ramunas Kondratas, then assistant curator at the National Museum of American History, Division of Medical Science at the Smithsonian Institution, made a rather unique documentary film on homeopathy. Featuring Gustav "Gus" Tafel, who took the audience on a 30-minute tour of the largest manufacturer of homeopathic medicines in the United States, Boericke & Tafel, "Reunions: Memories of an American Experience" presented a distinguished looking gentleman in his late sixties, the grandson of co-founder Adolph J. Tafel, who waxed nostalgic over his time at the "B & T" firm. Located in Philadelphia at 1011 Arch Street, the building, apparatus, and manufacturing processes had changed little since moving to that location in 1880.* The Skinner potencies† used by B & T until 1991, for example, had been recommended by the eminent homeopath James Tyler Kent in 1903, and even Gus Tafel admitted that many of the bottles of assorted attenuated and diluted tinctures made by that process had been lining the storage shelves for years.

But what exactly *is* homeopathy? The film's narrator explained that homeopathy was "a vitalistic and holistic medical doctrine formulated by a German physician, Samuel Hahnemann" in the early nineteenth century. After reviewing the company's history, Tafel toured the facility, introduced the audience to the firm's president (a "second cousin by marriage"), discussed the business through the years, and concluded with almost fatalistic resignation, "it [homeopathy] lasted until about 1900 and then it slowly started to deteriorate and then the allopathic schools took over." Happy with his B & T career, Tafel gave a wry

*In 1987 Boericke & Tafel was purchased by VSM in Holland. B & T moved in 1992 to Santa Rosa, California.

†Named after Scottish homeopath Thomas Skinner, the "Skinner Continuous Fluxion Apparatus" used by B & T was designed to produce highly dynamized products.

smile and reflected, "I won't say all the people were cured with the medicine they took, but it certainly didn't hurt 'em any and they never went after us on any kind of suit." The documentary ends by the narrator summing up with, "Homeopathy . . . is a link to another time. The future of this form of medicine is uncertain but it has a definite place in history."

True enough, and now at last we have a history told by America's most preeminent historian of alternative medicine, John S. Haller, Jr. Yet this film was mentioned for a definite reason. Anyone viewing this documentary would conclude that homeopathy in the United States was an ossified, nearly moribund alternative health system based upon a few notions concocted by an anachronistic German eccentric now carried on by a handful of kindly old men more from habit than conviction. The principles of like-cures-like and minuscule dose with its distinguishing potentized remedies appear quaint and well intentioned but hardly the things of which modern medicines are made. The book in hand, a sequel to *The History of Homeopathy: The Academic Years, 1820-1935* (2005), will quickly dispel this impressionistic view. Rather than presenting the picture of a slowly dying monolithic form of alternative medicine, John Haller demonstrates that homeopathy has fostered a multiplicity of beliefs and therapeutic modalities. Instead of the dry and dusty nooks and crannies of a struggling, superannuated homeopathic manufacturer, the present volume shows homeopathy to be a highly animated and constantly changing alternative to medical and even religious orthodoxy. Rather than the nearly expired profession bemoaned by Gus Tafel, we see here, as stated in the book's subtitle, homeopathy transitioning *From Rational Medicine to Holistic Health Care.* It is a lively narrative of conflict and controversy, carried up to the present day by a colorful cast of ever evolving and always interesting characters.

As Haller tells it, "In fact, classical homeopathy was anything but steady-state. As will eventually be shown, having wedded themselves to high potency therapeutics, classical homeopaths moved inexorably from an empirically grounded science to a religiously based belief system sporting a myriad of competing interpretations." Indeed the definition given in the documentary, namely, that homeopathy is a "vitalistic and holistic medical doctrine," is broadly true but in the search for more spiritual cures the devil has always been in the details. The book in hand demonstrates that there have been almost as many views of homeopathy as there have been homeopaths. These diverse perspectives form a kaleidoscope of theories and regimens—everything from Swedenborgianism-turned-Kentianism to Reichenbach's "Odic force" theory have produced an array of therapies from Electronic Attentuator X-O-Rays, Schüssler's cell-salts, and Bach flowerism to high potencies, low potencies, somewhere-in-between potencies, and other so-called energy medicines—all (or at least most) formulated under the homeopathic shibboleth of *similia similibus curantur* or (as some have insisted) *similia similibus curentur.*

As complicated as all this sounds, Haller gives insight, strength, and clarity to this story by allowing the protagonists to speak for themselves. In less competent hands such a cacophony of voices would become a hodgepodge of atonality, losing the narrative and the reader in an anarchy of sound bites. But through Haller's seasoned expertise and objective analysis homeopathy's search for itself, though persistently elusive, still emerges with verve and precision. Thoroughly researched and drawn from the primary sources themselves, *The History of American Homeopathy: From Rational Medicine to Holistic Health Care* forms the second volume of what will undoubtedly become the standard history of this heterodox system of health care in the United States.

Despite the story's complexity, Haller's theme is straightforward: with the decline of the academic years following the Flexner Report in 1910, a growing laity emerged as the heir apparent to the system founded by Samuel Hahnemann nearly two centuries ago. Yet even sailing under this new populist banner has remained problematic. Haller admits, ". . . whether American homeopathy can ever share in conventional medicine's broad-based integration remains to be seen. Having moved so far into the world of the non-professional healer and having thereby distanced itself from most licensure requirements tied to training, testing, and certification, whether homeopathy can be anything more than a faith-based system dependent upon anecdotes, beliefs, theories, preconceived notions, testimonials and opinions of support is questionable. Ultimately, this may be what its proponents have wanted all along."

In the final analysis the history of homeopathy has been anything but homogeneous and this has plagued its historiography. Too often the history of homeopathy has been chronicled by extremists—crusaders out to vilify it as unmitigated quackery or partisan apologists and thinly veiled hagiographers eager to justify nearly everything and/or anything in its name. This is no such volume. Haller lets homeopathy explain itself, and in so doing a fascinating history emerges. The following chapters tell a story that is multifaceted, diverse, and sometimes contentious but *never* boring.

Michael A. Flannery
Professor and Associate Director for Historical Collections
Lister Hill Library of the Health Sciences
University of Alabama at Birmingham

Acknowledgments

Those to whom I am indebted include Michael A. Flannery, Professor and Associate Director for Historical Collections, Lister Hill Library of the Health Sciences, University of Alabama at Birmingham, for his years of steady support and encouragement; Dennis B. Worthen, Scholar in Residence at the Lloyd Library and Museum in Cincinnati; Pascal James Imperato, MD, Professor and Founding Dean, School of Public Health at the State University of New York Health Science Center at Brooklyn; Christopher Hoolihan, Head of Rare Books and Manuscripts at the Edward G. Minor Library at the University of Rochester Medical Center; Director Maggie Heran and staff members Carol Maxwell, Betsy Kruthoffer, Anna Heran, Jan Mueller, and Heather Newkirk of the Lloyd Library and Museum; librarians Kathy Fahey, Mary K. Taylor, David Koch, Barbara Preece, Kimbra Stout, and David Carlson of Morris Library, Southern Illinois University, Carbondale; curator Barbara Mason of the Pearson Museum; librarian Connie Poole and staff from the Southern Illinois University School of Medicine Library in Springfield, Illinois; librarian Deirdre Clarkin and staff at the National Library of Medicine; executive assistant Marie Antoinette Moyers in the Office of the President at Southern Illinois University; and the librarians and support staff of the Newberry Library; Johns Hopkins University Library; Ohio State University Library; Yale Medical Library; University of Chicago Library; the Widener Library of Harvard University; University of California Library, Davis; Flower Veterinary Library of Cornell University; Health Sciences Library of the University of Washington; National College of Naturopathic Medicine; John Hay Library of Brown University; Kent State University Library; University of Maryland Library; New York State Library, Albany; Historical Society of Pennsylvania; Meadville Theological

Library; and the Theodore Lownik Library of Illinois Benedictine College.

As always, I am grateful to my wife Robin, who offered inspiration, encouragement, criticism, and substantial assistance, including the reading of drafts and indexing the finished manuscript.

The History of American Homeopathy

Introduction

A medical system more diverse than modern homeopathy is almost unimaginable. The multiplicity of its beliefs makes it difficult to decide whether it is a single healing system or a plural system supporting multiple practices. This complexity of character has been a part of homeopathy's leitmotif since its founding but is more prominent now than ever before. Today, there is no single perspective in homeopathic theory and practice; nor is there any one preeminent authority—canonical or heretical. Like modern Christianity, which can and does accommodate such extremes as monasticism, televangelism, Appalachian snake handlers, exorcism, incantations, and liberation theology, homeopathy has flourished by accommodating to the needs of its many disciples with myriad beliefs and practices. Low and high energy medicines; the single remedy method common to the British Isles, the United States and South America; the system of polypharmacy common in France and Germany; the Indian preference for hypodermic water infusion and for visualizing the organism in etheric layers; and the variances between and among constitutional typologies, individualization, and the doctrine of signatures—all have found a home within homeopathy's varied modalities and cultures. In some ways modern homeopathy is more eclectic than its historical nemesis, conventional medicine.

This book represents a continuation of *The History of American Homeopathy: The Academic Years, 1820-1936,* published by Haworth in 2005.

Chapter 1 ("The Decline of Academic Homeopathy") recounts the origins of homeopathy's medical education system, its long-standing goal to become a specialty within conventional medicine, the sobering sense of betrayal felt by conservatives as its schools moved beyond

Hahnemann's principles, and the closing of its remaining colleges, hospitals, and clinics in the 1920s and 1930s.

Chapter 2 ("Esoteric Homeopathy") describes the unbridled theories that proliferated in the wake of academic homeopathy's demise in the late nineteenth and early twentieth centuries, their relationship to homeopathy's vitalistic underpinnings, the alliance forged between physical healing and the higher spiritual planes, and the emergence of homeopathy as a "belief" system distinct from science.

Chapter 3 ("The Laity Speaks Out") traces the growth of the laity as a force within homeopathy, their outspoken adherence to Hahnemann's original principles, their rejection of all forms of adjectival medicine, and their growing role in the practice of domestic homeopathy offsetting the decline in trained homeopathic physicians.

Chapter 4 ("Postwar Trends") explains the expansion of homeopathy in the aftermath of the Second World War, its links during the late 1950s and early 1960s with Eastern philosophies, the growth of psychosomatic medicine, and homeopathy's steady move away from rational medical science toward a more cultist and metaphysical view of healing.

Chapter 5 ("Roads Taken and Not Taken") identifies the challenges homeopathy faced as the ranks of its medically educated physicians were replaced by increasing numbers of unlicensed lay practitioners, the struggle within homeopathy's associations over membership credentials, and the long-term implications of homeopathy's change in status to that of a nonmedical therapy.

Chapter 6 ("Whither the Future?") highlights the controversy between and among homeopaths as to whether their leaders had gone too far in their acceptance of new ideas, thus forsaking homeopathy's classical roots, or whether the more speculative elements of their belief system as professed by its nonmedically trained professionals are consistent with Hahnemann's original vision.

Unlike its European counterpart, American homeopathy advocated a more spiritual or metaphysical view of healing that repudiated reductionist science and its gold standard of randomized double-blind clinical trials—thus preventing it from garnering a place within mainstream medicine. Its thinly veiled vitalism conceived of a universe reduced to a single set of governing principles and envisioned the body's health not only attuned to a higher reality, but also sustained through interaction between the material and spiritual dimensions of life.

It is this spiritual dimension that Andrew Weil, MD, clinical professor of internal medicine and director of the Program in Integrative Medicine at the University of Arizona in Tucson, finds deficient in conventional medicine today. Unlike the homeopath, chiropractor, or Chinese acupuncturist who can elaborate on the state of the body's balance, on symptom patterns, or life energy and universal forces, conventional medical doctors seem either unable or unconcerned to enunciate any coherent philosophy. Schooled in a materialistic and reductionist learning environment, the graduates of the nation's regular medical schools seem unable or unwilling to factor nonmaterial determinants into health and disease. Thus, for Weil, author of the popular *Health and Healing* (1983), such concepts as "belief," "thought," "emotion," and "spiritual force," which are key elements in unconventional medicine, are little more than fictions that, lacking in scientific relevance, have little or no bearing in medicine. This "professional blindness," he explains, keeps conventional medicine from appreciating the "mental" side of health and healing.[1]

Weil's criticism, however, may be too one-sided. Unlike alternative healing systems that fear being lost in any integration with conventional health care, regular medicine is today less inclined to condemn those who disagree with it or who offer differing points of view. Indeed, spiritual and psychological factors such as "emotional care," "suggestion," "empathy," "relaxation," "meditation," and "prayer" have long been acknowledged as having a role in the healing equation though not factorable in evidence-based medicine. Arguably there is a greater sense of tolerance today than ever before of concepts related to self-healing. This openness may be explained by the high cost of conventional medicine which drives the search for less costly interventions. I am inclined to believe, however, that it is also due to a persistent willingness among regular physicians to expect the unexpected. For this reason, many complementary healing systems are welcomed for their contributions to the therapeutic encounter.[2]

Whether American homeopathy can ever share in conventional medicine's broad-based integration remains to be seen. Having moved so far into the world of the nonprofessional healer and having thereby distanced itself from most licensure requirements tied to training, testing, and certification, whether homeopathy can be anything more than a faith-based system dependent upon anecdotes, beliefs, theories, preconceived notions, testimonials, and opinions of support is questionable. Ultimately, this may be what its proponents have wanted all along.

Chapter 1

The Decline of Academic Homeopathy

Reflecting on the history of academic homeopathy from 1850 to roughly 1900, and its precipitous decline thereafter, homeopathic authors Daniel Cook, MD, and Alain Naudé sought in an article published in 1996 to dispel the widespread belief that this earlier period represented the "Golden Age" of homeopathy in America. What had once appeared as "promising and bright," they explained, was not homeopathy at all, but rather "a caricature of homeopathy" that neither Abraham Flexner in his classic *Medical Education in the United States and Canada* (1910) nor the American Medical Association were responsible for creating. Instead, homeopathy had collapsed because "the vast majority of those who called themselves homeopaths lacked integrity." With too few qualified teachers in its medical colleges, and having decided to emulate orthodox medical education rather than structure schools along the lines of its early Allentown Academy, homeopathic education had become a mere reflection of conventional medicine, borrowing freely its concepts, diagnoses, and treatments. With single remedies denounced and potentized remedies rejected, and with the Law of Similia similarly discarded, little remained of true homeopathy. "Students at American homeopathic colleges between 1850 and 1900," reasoned the authors, "were taught to examine patients allopathically, diagnose allopathically, and then treat these allopathic conceptions of disease with any and every homeopathic, allopathic, and herbal drug having a reputation for getting rid of the pathological 'entity' they diagnosed." Thus, in the so-called Golden Age of homeopathy, very few of Samuel Hahnemann's (1755-1843) principles were taught or practiced by the physicians who graduated from its schools. Instead, homeopathy was overrun by eclectics and other pseudo-healers who falsely represented themselves as trained homeopaths. That homeopathy did not die completely was due to the perseverance of a small band of purists, many of whom were laypersons, who slowly but steadily captured lost ground to become the "voice" of a new and truer homeopathy.[1]

This revisionist history was further reinforced several years later by Julian Winston, author of *Faces of Homeopathy* (1999), who explained that homeopathy's medical schools were teaching conventional medicine with a "smattering" of homeopathic therapeutics mixed in. Trained in name but not in practice, the faculties of these schools had "slipped further and further into 'expediency' " while continuing to call themselves homeopaths. By the 1920s, explained Winston, "homeopathy's façade was barely standing."[2]

These interpretations allowed homeopaths to blame their troubles on the trustees and faculty of their failing colleges rather than on a host of competing heresies that consumed homeopathy during those same years. The revisionist interpretations also presumed that at the core of their reform movement a small group of believers held fast to something called *classical* homeopathy. These believers included conservatives within the American Institute of Homeopathy (AIH) (founded in 1844), dedicated purists who formed the International Hahnemannian Association (IHA) in 1880, and disenchanted laypersons who had held firm to Hahnemann's principles and who would later help establish the American Foundation for Homeopathy (AFH) in 1921.[3] While these ratiocinations provide a self-serving and useful interpretation of homeopathy as it emerged out of the Flexner years, they ignored what in fact was a much more complicated set of events. To be sure, they gave credence to the victory of the so-called classicists over the progressive wing of homeopathy and, in the process, allowed the victors the luxury of writing themselves into posterity. However, history is not always what the victors say it is, and in this case, these representative authors chose to ignore not only a major transformation in the art and science of medicine but also significant feuds and variances within homeopathic theory and practice.

THE "HOLY GRAIL"

The *Nordamerikanische Akademie der homöopathischen Heilkunst* (North American Academy of the Homeopathic Art) in Allentown, Pennsylvania, incorporated by the Pennsylvania Legislature on June 17, 1836, was the first homeopathic medical college in the world. Structured on the concept of postgraduate education, its curriculum consisted of lectures offered during the summer months when regular medical schools were not in session. The faculty's goal was to make homeopathy a legitimate option or specialty within regular medicine. Over time, the pursuit of this option trumped all other objectives, becoming the "holy grail" of the AIH, the first successful national association of medical doctors and parent to a host of state and county societies. Despite this objective, the burden of persecution by regulars who vigorously opposed legitimizing homeopathy forced the reformers into organizing free-standing homeopathic medical colleges offering a full curriculum. When this occurred, the specialty or postgraduate objective was laid aside as homeopaths set out to replicate old school curricula. By the turn of the twentieth century, American homeopaths were supporting twenty-two schools in fourteen different states.[4] With the exception of the Allentown Academy which closed in 1842, all subsequent homeopathic colleges operated as mirror images of allopathic institutions, teaching the same subjects except for therapeutics and materia medica.[5]

To complicate matters even more, medical doctors in both Europe and America were deeply influenced by the work of the French Clinical School, with the result that medical education began a long and arduous migration toward a more empirically based medical science. The diaspora of ideas and statistically based research emanating from the French hospitals not only affected mainstream medicine, but also touched the thinking of homeopaths at home and abroad. European homeopaths reveled in these new currents of thinking and quietly incorporated them within the context of their sectarian ideas. In doing so, they garnered toleration from mainstream medicine which eventually opened its doors to homeopathy as a specialty.

The same was true within the progressive wing of American homeopathy. Following the discoveries of Gabriel Andral (1797-1876), Pierre C. A. Louis (1787-1872), Jean Baptist Bouillaud (1796-1881),

Pierre Adolphe Piorry (1794-1879), Léon Rostan (1790-1866), and others of the Paris Clinical School, American homeopaths moved quickly to adapt new clinical techniques and teaching practices, and new modes of organizing medical knowledge. Decades later, this same wing would join in celebrating the discoveries of Louis Pasteur (1822-1895) and Robert Koch (1843-1910) in germ theory and move assertively to incorporate more modern diagnostic procedures, biochemistry, serologic, endocrinologic, vaccine, and other pharmacological agents into their medicine. For them, it was essential "to be up to date in all that pertains to therapeutics" so that homeopathists could add to their efficiency as physicians. Bacteriology had been of great value to allopathic medicine and to progressive homeopaths and their therapeutic practices as well.[6]

Nevertheless, American homeopathy remained divided: while the progressive wing chose to use the medical school curriculum as its vehicle for change, the conservative wing chose to chase the high-potency beliefs of its more metaphysical proponents. Thus, two broad classes of homeopaths came to exist, each differing as to the terms and conditions of what Hahnemann stood for as well as his methods of practice. One class wanted homeopathy to follow the course of medicine as it moved from rational system-building to empirical science; the other held that homeopathy was a therapeutic system with exclusive principles, rules, and methods that were as unchanging as Newton's law of gravitation.[7] This latter group interpreted classical homeopathy as something it never was, namely a composite of unchanging principles and practices. In fact, classical homeopathy was anything but steady state. As will eventually be shown, having wedded themselves to high-potency therapeutics, classical homeopaths moved inexorably from an empirically grounded science to a religiously based belief system sporting myriad competing interpretations.

THE HIGH-POTENCY CONSERVATIVES

Conservative homeopaths, also called Hahnemannians, grew increasingly alarmed as the graduates of their colleges showed a marked preference for the lower potencies rather than those more attenuated, and who had more or less assimilated the newer findings coming out of the Paris Clinical School into their theory and practice. This concern most troubled J. A. Ward, MD, of New York who, at the sixteenth annual session of the AIH in 1859, accused his progressive colleagues of pretending to be believers in the homeopathic law, but who actually ridiculed and condemned the teachings of Hahnemann and his "Heaven born system." In Ward's opinion, these "nondescripts" were busy merging homeopathy into the pernicious mazes of allopathy, eclecticism, and other empirical schools.[8]

Bitter fighting between the conservative and progressive wings of homeopathy continued into the post-Civil War decades as, increasingly, academic pedagogy moved in the direction of clinical and laboratory-based medicine. At the twenty-third session of the AIH which opened in Chicago on June 6, 1870, Carroll Dunham, MD (1828-1887), of the New York Homeopathic Medical College spoke on the subject of "Freedom of Medical Opinion and Action, a Vital Necessity and a Great Responsibility." In his remarks, Dunham challenged the membership to perform as "true homeopaths" or move on. While he did not advocate exclusion of those who refused to accept the strict creed of homeopathy, he urged the AIH to establish "an unquestionable therapeutic system, or law, for the guidance of every practitioner under the standard of Hahnemann."[9] These feelings were echoed by David Dyce Brown, MD, in his *The Reign of Law in Medicine* (1886) who thought it presumptuous to question any of Hahnemann's theories. Hahnemann was "worthy of the greatest genius, and he has literally left nothing for his disciples to do but carry out his principles."[10] Arthur G. Allen, MD, of Philadelphia was even more definitive. Homeopathy stood forth as a positive science, a "rock of truth, as never-changing as the universe itself."[11]

Not surprisingly, the tension between progressive and conservative elements in homeopathy did not lapse in the ensuing years. In an effort to rectify the consequences of this split and halt the trend toward greater liberality, conservatives established the International Hahnemannian Association (IHA) in 1880 to advance the teachings of strict Hahnemannianism in medical therapeutics, that is, symptomatology, single remedies, high dilutions, and applying the Law of Similia universally based on the principles taught by Hahnemann in his *Organon of the Healing* Art (1833).[12] The high-potency advocates who formed the IHA were the metaphysical followers of Hahnemann who dedicated themselves to keeping alive the letter and spirit of what they termed classical homeopathy. Through the IHA's bureaus of homeopathic philosophy, materia medica, and clinical medicine, its members set out to demonstrate that homeopathy still had a name to defend and principles to maintain—principles laid down by Hahnemann himself in the *Organon.* Their ideal was "pure homeopathy, nothing more, nothing less."[13]

In the fall of 1890, a group of prominent Hahnemannians arranged a charter for the Philadelphia Post-Graduate School of Homeopathics. The object of the school was to teach pure homeopathy as the universal application in disease using the 1833 edition of Hahnemann's *Organon.* This included the single remedy in the single dose in the minimum quantity; a combination of didactic and clinical instruction; renewed emphasis in the seven distinct departments of materia medica and the philosophy of homeopathy; clinical medicine with focus on diseases of women and children, obstetrics, and diseases of the eye and ear; and surgery.[14] Despite good intentions, the school failed to maintain itself as a distinctive representative of Hahnemannian philosophy and practice, due in part to an infusion of Swedenborgian doctrines (see Chapter 2) into the system of homeopathy, thereby giving the instruction a religious and theological character more so than a scientific and empirical basis. Its graduates were of high quality, but few if any joined ranks in supporting and maintaining the school. Nevertheless, the Hahnemannians continued to pursue the idea of postgraduate training as the answer to their critique of the colleges.[15]

Soon after the Philadelphia Post-Graduate School of Homeopathics was established, the Hering Medical College was founded in Chicago in 1892 as the outgrowth of the "compromising attitude" assumed by other homeopathic colleges.[16] Established as a protest against those graduates who had left their respective alma maters "without true knowledge, without enthusiasm, and without faith in their methods," Hering Medical College took as its basis the principles of the *Organon.* It promised to offer a course of lectures equivalent to the leading colleges of medicine and also provide systematic and comprehensive training in advanced materia medica and therapeutics and the philosophy of homeopathy. Its library was adorned with more than three hundred colored engravings of medicinal plants and within the college was Hering Institute, a fraternity whose object was the social, intellectual, and scientific advancement of its members. Another feature of the college was its connection to neighboring hospitals including the Chicago Baptist Hospital, National Temperance Hospital, Women's Christian Temperance Union Hospital, and Cook County Hospital. The college also had access to laboratories built by the University of Chicago devoted to botany, zoology, anatomy, and physiology.[17] In 1903, Hering Medical College affiliated with Dunham Medical College, making it the strongest school in the teaching of classical homeopathy.

Notwithstanding these efforts, conservatives bewailed the fact that their beloved system was disappearing as their members dwindled and their hospitals lost accreditation. The editor of the *Pacific Coast Journal of Homeopathy* blamed the AIH for the short-sighted policy of its Council on Medical Education and the remaining homeopathic journals for their lack of "rugged individuality." For the editor of the *Homeopathic Recorder,* the "stereotyped, cut-and-dried" policies of the AIH had unwittingly contributed to these problems. In attempting to make homeopathy a "system" of medicine rather than a therapeutic specialty, the AIH had encouraged homeopathy to spread itself over the entire field of medicine—a challenge it failed to accomplish.[18]

EDUCATIONAL STANDARDS

What conservative homeopaths failed to appreciate was that by the 1890s, minimum standards for practicing medicine had been established in twenty-nine states supporting a population of 41,000,000 people. States in which the license displaced the diploma included Alabama, Minnesota, Mississippi, Montana, New Jersey, New York, North Carolina, North Dakota, South Carolina, Virginia, and Washington, as well as the Indian Territory (Cherokee Nation). The states where supervision of the diploma was established either by health or examining boards, or by censors of state medical societies included California, Colorado, Delaware, Florida, Illinois, Iowa, Kentucky, Missouri, Nebraska, New Hampshire, New Mexico, Oregon, South Dakota, Tennessee, Vermont, and West Virginia, as well as the Indian Territory (Choctaw Nation).[19]

The raising of standards was not without complications for homeopaths since the legislation creating state examining and licensing boards gave a clear majority to mainstream or regular medicine. These reforms were advocated as a method for elevating the standards of medical education and diminishing the number of unqualified practitioners. Homeopaths were justifiably concerned, however, that other less savory objectives were also intended. For this reason, they took issue with any "compulsory union" of legally recognized and incorporated schools of medicine. The single board, they surmised, was a "cunning device" to destroy homeopathy as a distinct sect, make old school doctors the legal censors of medical education, and force a "perpetual brand of inferiority" on applicants from sectarian schools."[20] According to C. E. Walton, MD, of Cincinnati, the *only* single board beyond suspicion was one composed of equal numbers of allopathic, homeopathic, and eclectic physicians who confined their examination to anatomy, physiology, pathology, histology, chemistry, surgery, midwifery, and posology, but not materia medica or therapeutics.[21] However, homeopathy's preferred structure was that which had been established in New York where the legislature created three separate boards of medical examiners, each representing a distinct school of practice. As a result, the law gave no preference for any system to the exclusion of any other.[22]

By 1900, the AIH was facing mounting pressure from its more conservative members to return to the original principles and practices of Hahnemann. Indicative of this were comments made in homeopathic journals that any future president of the AIH must be "a homeopath of the homeopaths, a recognized leader proud of his principles and prepared to defend them, a man to whom every homeopathic physician can point as a representative man of the school."[23] Nevertheless, the lines were drawn between the proponents of scientific homeopathy and the champions of strict Hahnemannianism as it seemed that neither group could agree on a common set of principles.[24] Some found fault with the materia medica and were convinced that it was necessary to take the entire homeopathic inventory of drugs through a reproving, especially those potencies above the 12th attenuation. There were those who felt that all practices should be carried out only with high potencies while still others preferred low dilutions, alternating remedies, and combination tablets. There were even those who favored patent medicines and supplementary nonhomeopathic regimens. Besides these differences, homeopaths were also divided on whether to treat by way of the disease name or by the symptom-complex, and whether to use or abandon the repertory. According to William L. Morgan, MD, of Baltimore, barely 5 percent of the homeopathic physicians in the United States actually practiced according to the principles of their founder.[25]

Those homeopaths who practiced a mixed system were called "mongrels" or "mixers" by their conservative opponents. The same sobriquets were applied to the colleges. By 1900, the sectarian character of homeopathic colleges had begun to dramatically lessen as more progressive trustees and faculty struggled to incorporate the implications of germ theory and the newer laboratory sciences. Most schools professed and even advertised an "adjectival" homeopathy, meaning that they taught and practiced a modified or more progressive form of medicine.[26] Among progressives, the college curriculum was neither long enough nor thorough enough; the materia medica was not scientific enough; provings lacked completeness; clinical symptoms were recklessly unreliable; and the literature no longer seemed relevant.[27] As further evidence of these impediments, progressives pointed to a steady exodus of students from their colleges to those of allopathy. "It is idle to dispute the fact that this [migration] is constantly increasing," admitted one concerned physician. The motivation for it was the dissatisfaction of students with what they perceived as obsolete instruction. "They grow weary of the constant harking back a hundred years for therapeutic teachings," he remarked. The younger generation of physicians demanded scientific accuracy and, while the allopathic colleges offered little more than "therapeutic quicksand," they nonetheless introduced students to the rigors of modern science.[28]

Of course, the embarrassment perceived by progressive students and faculty was the very source of Hahnemannian pride and the raison d'etre for the colleges in the first place. Critics like William L. Morgan believed that the very accommodations made by faculty and trustees to comply with state licensing standards were the root of the problem. Now, very few students were actually studying Hahnemann's *Organon* in their courses; at best, the book was only tangentially mentioned in lectures. In the announcements of nine medical colleges, Morgan found only two that provided courses on the *Organon,* and only one of these was taught by a full-time faculty member. He concluded that in most homeopathic schools, that which distinguished them from allopathic colleges was simply the word homeopathy on their circulars. Believing that the *Organon* stood in the same relation to therapeutics as arithmetic did to mathematics or as grammar to language, he urged that the book once again become the anchor in all instruction. Only when students had read and thoroughly studied the *Organon,* the system of chronic diseases, and the use of the repertory and materia medica, could they be considered capable of practicing homeopathy as it was intended. Only then would they be able to manage the life and health of their patients without resorting to the subterfuges of narcotics, coal oil derivatives, antitoxins, serum and hypodermic treatment, and local treatments of any kind. Only then could the physician honestly be judged for what he professed.[29]

Morgan urged college trustees to provide greater oversight of the curriculum, ensuring that the faculty was capable of teaching homeopathic philosophy and its applications in the various branches. Teachers should first understand what Hahnemann wrote and taught before undertaking "to reform what Hahnemann did." In teaching the *Organon,* Morgan advocated special emphasis be given to the spirit-like vital force that animated the body. This force affected both the disease and the drug. The drug, as material matter, was inert, but it possessed a subtle and active vitality that gave it features different from all other material substances. This vital theory of disease genesis as opposed to the organic germ theory of allopathic medicine constituted homeopathy's distinguishing character. Admitting that this drug action, known as the Law of Similia, was no better understood than gravitation, chemical affinity, or electricity, Morgan nonetheless insisted that it served the cause of medicine in the most important and essential way.[30]

THE FLEXNER REPORT AND ITS AFTERMATH

In 1908, the Carnegie Foundation for the Advancement of Teaching authorized a comparison of medical education in the United States and Canada with that of Great Britain, Germany, and France. Concerned that medical education had become a commercialized institution and had deteriorated to the point where patients could make little distinction between the well-trained and poorly trained physician,

Henry S. Pritchett, president of the foundation, appointed Abraham Flexner (1866-1959), a graduate of Johns Hopkins and a renowned schoolmaster in Louisville to carry out the study. Flexner visited each of the 155 existing schools, including fifteen homeopathic, eight eclectic, eight osteopathic, and one physio-medical college. Although his visits seldom lasted more than one or two days, Flexner had little difficulty in abstracting the information needed for his investigation. More often than not, he discovered schools that were not much more than commercial enterprises under the control of cliques of local doctors with little or no hospital connection. Like many progressive thinkers in his day, Flexner preferred social control to drift and was by no means reluctant to suggest the power of the state as an agent of reform.[31]

Assessing the strengths and weaknesses of the country's homeopathic schools, Flexner concluded that only Boston University School of Medicine, the New York Homeopathic Medical College and Flower Hospital, and the Hahnemann Medical College of Philadelphia were capable of teaching the fundamental branches of medicine. Although they lacked full-time instructors, their laboratories in anatomy, pathology, bacteriology, and physiology were sufficient. The remaining schools were either deficient in laboratory facilities or refused to acknowledge their relevance. Of the fifteen homeopathic schools, Flexner considered six to be "utterly hopeless." These included Southwestern Homeopathic Medical College in Louisville, Pulte Medical College in Cincinnati, Southern Homeopathic Medical College in Baltimore, Hering Medical College in Chicago, the Detroit Homeopathic College, and the Kansas City Homeopathic Medical College.[32]

George Royal (1853-1931), chair of the AIH's Council on Medical Education and professor of materia medica and therapeutics in the Homeopathic Medical Department at the State University of Iowa did not hesitate to accuse Flexner of being ill equipped for the job given him by the Carnegie Foundation, claiming that he was neither trained as a teacher nor as a practitioner of medicine. As a consequence, Flexner had done an injustice to patients and to scores of medical colleges, forcing medical teachers to neglect the art and the practical part of medicine in order to teach the science of medicine. "While I would not say that Mr. Flexner put too much stress upon the science of medicine," Royal quipped, "I do assert that he did not put nearly enough stress upon the art of medicine. His conception of medicine is neither clear, nor logical, nor symmetrical."[33] By contrast, the Boston University School of Medicine took righteous pride in Flexner's assessment and used his comments to its advantage in recruiting students. The school's dean, John P. Sutherland, made note of the report in his opening address to incoming students, referring to Flexner's praise of the school's laboratory and clinical facilities.[34]

It would be wrong to assume that the AIH was insensitive to the need for reform since its own Council on Medical Education had recommended raising the standards of medical education in general; securing the adoption of a uniform curriculum in all of its colleges; and securing the enactment of legislation that would deal justly with student, teacher, patient, and physician.[35] The council visited and inspected eighteen homeopathic, eclectic, and osteopathic schools in 1909, using a rating system adopted in 1907. Before beginning its inspections, the council visited several allopathic colleges for comparison. While all eighteen schools were extended "recognition" by the council, it was evident that not all was well. The Missouri College of Homeopathy of St. Louis suspended operations shortly after the council's visit and the board of regents of the University of Minnesota voted to abolish all but two chairs in its College of Homeopathic Medicine and Surgery.[36] Similarly, at the opening of the 1910-1911 session of the Hahnemann Medical College of Philadelphia, the dean announced a radical change in the curriculum for juniors and seniors. Following the model established by Johns Hopkins and Harvard, didactic lectures were reduced to a minimum and advanced students were directed to devote a greater amount of their time to practical clinical work in the hospital wards and in the outpatient department.[37]

In 1914, all homeopathic teaching institutions were placed under the supervision of the AIH and its Council on Medical Education. The council made no attempt to grade teaching institutions using a classification system; instead, it supervised entrance requirements, curricula, and general management of the ten remaining homeopathic medical schools to see that they functioned within the laws of the states wherein they were located. The council also engaged in the work of hospital inspection since graduates would soon be required to have at least one year of hospital residency for the diploma or a license to practice.[38] As chairman of the council, George Royal visited all the colleges and found the same conditions existing in varying degrees, namely, the reluctance to teach the *Organon.* Only Hering Medical College of Chicago was the exception.[39]

In 1911, homeopathy boasted 10 national societies, 5 regional societies, 35 state societies, 101 local societies, 49 clubs, 8 college alumni associations, 4 miscellaneous associations, 60 hospitals, 38 mixed hospitals, 13 colleges, and 20 journals.[40] By 1916, there was one less national society, two fewer regional societies, three fewer state societies, twenty fewer local societies, three fewer medical colleges, and two fewer medical journals.[41] Of the nine homeopathic colleges that remained in 1918, five were coeducational, and one was exclusively for women. All met the requirements of the Federation of State Medical Boards of the United States and were on the accredited list of colleges of that organization. However, the higher standards of the AMA's Council of Medical Education rated five of the schools as Class "A," three as Class "B," and one as Class "C." Convinced that there was no discrimination, G. M. Cushing, MD, of Chicago urged all homeopathic colleges to upgrade to Class "A" or close. "There is only one excuse for the existence of any medical college today, be it homeopathic or regular," he advised, "and that is the production of a superior type of doctor." Unless that can be done, "there is no excuse for our existence as a separate school and the money now used for carrying on of our colleges can best be diverted into other channels and the students sent to institutions where they will be better trained."[42]

In 1918, the Boston University School of Medicine added a chair of Old School materia medica and therapeutics. The action was significant in that it meant the college would no longer have to register as sectarian, since mainstream therapeutics was now taught in conjunction with homeopathic therapeutics. That same year, the Hahnemann Medical College of the Pacific amalgamated with the University of California although its Department of Applied Homeopathy was retained in the organizational change.[43] A year later, the college's hospital passed into the hands of the university.[44] Also on March 28, 1919, House Bill No. 454 was signed into law establishing a Department of Homeopathic Materia Medica and Therapeutics in the State University of Iowa, replacing its College of Homeopathic Medicine.[45]

Thomas J. Preston, dean of New York Homeopathic Medical College and Flower Hospital, lamented the fact that in 1919 only six colleges remained, with fewer than 100 graduating annually. In his estimation, the seeds of homeopathy's educational malaise stemmed from the lack of research carried out as part of the life of the colleges. "We should have more research work done in our colleges because it helps to keep the spirit of the student alive," he wrote. Even if this meant fewer colleges, Preston favored the move provided it meant achieving Class "A" status. The colleges must teach the principles of homeopathy, "but first and foremost, teach scientific medicine." The time for "ultra-sectarianism," he argued, had long since passed.[46]

For Claude A. Burrett, MD, dean of the College of Homeopathic Medicine at Ohio State University, the program's lack of a strong research base had proved particularly frustrating. In an article entitled "Modern Medical Education" and published in the *Journal of the American Institute of Homeopathy (JAIH),* he wrote about the discoveries of Pasteur; the advent of the science of bacteriology; and the budding new field of preventive medicine. He stressed the urgency of developing fully equipped laboratories and providing a solid foundation in chemistry, physics, and biology. "The hour has struck for medical progress," he wrote. "Will our homeopathic profession seize its opportunity?"[47]

In 1921, after the Homeopathic Department in the University of Michigan had declined to only forty-seven students, President Marion LeRoy Burton, worrying over the cost of unnecessary duplication, recommended the amalgamation of its regular and homeopathic schools. Dean Wilbert B. Hinsdale of the homeopathic department urged the state's homeopaths not to oppose the merger, but many of the faithful were outraged by the university's action. Their efforts, however, failed to reverse the decision.[48] When the college closed, only two postgraduate courses in homeopathy remained in the curriculum, one in the principles of homeopathy, the other in drug action.[49]

Similar events took place at Ohio University when President W. O. Thomson explained that the decision to discontinue the Homeopathic School of Medicine was made "not because of dissatisfaction with the operation of the college or of the hospital, or because of the unsatisfactory quality of the students, but rather because of the persistent opposition to homeopathy as a school of medicine." He concluded that, in future years, none but the dominant school could "enjoy the privileges of state support."[50] Shortly afterwards, the Alumni Association of Hahnemann Medical College of Chicago voted to make its alma mater nonsectarian. How much homeopathy would remain in the curriculum was left undecided. The resolution presented by the committee required a compulsory course in homeopathy but the alumni, in an obvious sign of indifference, refused to set the number of hours.[51]

At the 1922 annual meeting of the AIH, delegates heard a report from its Council on Medical Education that sounded almost like a requiem. The report concluded that the only salvation for homeopathy's colleges and for homeopathy itself lay in the support of its independent colleges and the severing of all ties with state universities. In Iowa, the state university had failed to provide a professor for the chairs of homeopathy, materia medica, and therapeutics. Nor had the school registered a single student in the program. With roughly 9,000 homeopaths in the United States, and with 174 having died during the year while only 62 graduated, the implications were ominous. The council hoped that a genuine postgraduate college could be established in Chicago or New York and financed by the profession.[52]

Most sectarian colleges failed to make the transition into Class "A" schools and, by the mid-1920s, the public had come to agree with Abraham Flexner that modern medicine had displaced sectarian medicine and its single-minded therapeutic methods. Besides public opinion, a deciding number of homeopaths—both conservatives and progressives—had come to the conclusion that having fewer homeopathic colleges where the whole four years' course was taken, or having postgraduate colleges for undergraduates and licensed physicians were the only options available. As proof of the former, Hahnemann of Philadelphia was receiving nearly 700 applications for a mere sixty places; New York Homeopathic Medical College and Flower Hospital reported 400 more applications than could be accepted; while Boston University reported 60 more than it could accommodate. However, unless the number of graduates increased and homeopathy could be taught thoroughly and conscientiously, homeopaths would have to place their future in the hands of postgraduate colleges as a way of furthering their sectarian philosophy.[53] The problem with these two options was the paucity of physicians going forth from their studies to practice and teach the tenets of homeopathy.

Nevertheless, Rudolph F. Rabe of the New York Homeopathic Medical College concluded that pushing these options was the only real choice. Homeopathy "must either go forward, or cease to be an influence in the scientific world; she cannot stand still and hope to live."[54] According to Rabe, narrow sectarianism had disappeared from the medical profession and given way to a broader scientific outlook. "A narrow spirit," he explained, "has no place in any field of human endeavor, and most assuredly not in the field of medicine." While he wrote in defense of the three fundamental principles of homeopathy (similimum, single remedy, and minimum dose), he declared the theory of chronic diseases and the three miasms (psora, syphilis, and sycosis) as beliefs no longer shared by the majority of homeopaths, most of whom "pay no attention to it in practice." From the standpoint of practical therapeutics, he argued, there was good reason to doubt the purity of homeopathic treatment concerning any of the miasms. Rabe hoped for a return of an intelligent homeopathy that did not treat diseases but patients; that taught students to visualize patients and remedies so that these might be brought together; and to stop apologizing for homeopathy. Unless this was done, "homeopathy in the United States is doomed to extinction."[55]

MERGER

"The homeopathy of today is not the homeopathy of any edition of Hahnemann's *Organon* any more than the orthodox therapy of today is that of Sydenham or Cullen, or the surgery of today that of Ambrose Pare," explained progressive advocate Conrad Wesselhoeft (1884-1962) in 1926. A graduate of Harvard Medical College and teacher at Boston University Medical School, he saw no excuse for segregating homeopaths from the rest of the profession. Those who preferred to isolate themselves from "wholesome communion" with the larger profession were at odds with the free exchange of ideas. At question was not whether homeopathy any longer mattered, but how modern homeopathy should be taught. For Wesselhoeft, it was essential that a student be versed in the fundamental sciences of medicine and be familiar as well with the newest diagnostic procedures. Once the sciences had been mastered, then homeopathy could be introduced, but not until the third year of medical training. Only then was the student in a position to grasp its salient features. If introduced to homeopathy too early, the student was apt to receive "a distorted view of the subject, with the result that he overestimate[d] its sphere of applicability in practice, or he fail[ed] to harmonize it with his medical knowledge and reject[ed] it as being unintelligible and useless." Every student of homeopathy must be deeply involved in biochemistry, endocrinology, immunology, serology, and pharmacology, making use of all these sciences in harmony with homeopathic theory. As a teacher of homeopathy, Wesselhoeft found himself in a "perplexing state of affairs" given the fact that conservative Hahnemannians looked upon all modern conceptions of disease as "incompatible" with homeopathic principles.[56]

For E. Wallace MacAdam, editor of the decidedly progressive *JAIH*, homeopathy had been forced into becoming sectarian because of the bigotry and intolerance of allopathy. Its choice had also been aggravated by Hahnemann's own intolerance and egoism. That was because Hahnemann proposed "an entire revolution in medicine." In addition, homeopathy suffered because of the "religious fervor" that motivated so many of its believers. However, MacAdam insisted that homeopathy was a science, not a religion.[57] For progressives like himself, homeopathy had accomplished its work and the time had come to end its sectarianism. Believing firmly in homeopathic principles and that these principles would be better advanced by taking down the barriers between the two schools, he urged his colleagues to disband their organizations and fraternize with regulars.[58]

Linn J. Boyd, MD (b. 1895) of New York, author of *A Study of the Simile in Medicine* (1936), concluded that neither Hahnemann's theory of psora nor his theory of dosage had any bearing on modern homeopathy. Both were due to a fundamental lack of understanding of basic pathology. Boyd was particularly incensed with high-potency advocates who entered "realms of dilution where Hahnemann only peered and certainly never dared to enter." He was also convinced that the homeopathic materia medica was too "overburdened" with subjective symptomatology. What Hahneman gave to medicine was something much more important—the Law of Similia—not dose, not psora, not dynamization, not vital force, not human provings, and certainly not rejection or ridicule of coal tar derivatives and aspirin.[59]

During Boyd's editorship of the *JAIH*, the journal became a mirror of the thought and practice of the progressive school of homeopathic medicine. The fund of information swelled as the journal published scientific articles from European physicians and scientists. No longer was there a sense of inferiority as the *JAIH* published the lecture notes of Timothy Field Allen (1837-1902), professor of materia medica at New York Homeopathic Medical College and author of *Encyclopedia of Pure Materia Medica* (1874-79); the notes of Willis A. Dewey (1858-1938), co-author with William Boericke of *The Twelve Tissue Remedies of Schüssler* (1888); the published works of Karl Kotschau on natural methods of healing; the investigations on potencies by the University of Leningrad; selected writings of German pharmacologist Hugo Schulz (1853-1932), cofounder of the Arndt-Schulz phenomena; the works of Professor August Bier (1861-1949) who argued for greater respect of scientific homeopathy; and many articles on both clinical and experimental medicine. Also during Boyd's editorship, the journal became financially self-supporting due principally to improved business management and the acquisition of regular advertisers: Boericke and Runyon, Boericke and Tafel, Bristol-Myers Company; Carnrick and Company; Denver Chemical Company; Ehrhart and Karl, Inc.; Hahnemann Medical College; Horlick's Malted Milk Corp.; Lloyd Brothers; Kalak Water Company; Huxley Laboratories; Johnson and Johnson; Nestles Milk Products, Inc.; New York Homeopathic Medical College; Sharp and Dohme; E. R. Squibb and Sons; United Fruit Company; and Valentine's Meat Juice Company.

According to Boyd, homeopathy made more scientific progress in the late 1920s than in the previous sixty years. His comment was only partially self-serving. In looking at the index of the *JAIH,* it is clear that a new direction had been taken and, rather than pining over lost colleges, societies, and members, the journal had begun publishing articles addressing such subjects as constitutional factors in disease; the healing of wounds; assays of homeopathic tinctures; and lectures on materia medica, the homeopathic side of surgery, prenatal care, drugs effects, and natural healing. With "psychic causality" and "biologic causality" having now asserted themselves in medicine and with them the "teleologic" viewpoint, Boyd predicted that in the future, homeopathic literature would become increasingly more complex as well as more experimental. Such was the challenge ahead in experimental pharmacology. "The slogan of scientific medicine today," he reminded readers, "is not to hold ground won but to advance. This does not mean to discard the old but to incorporate the new."[60]

Boyd also took the opportunity to point out to fellow homeopaths that there was probably no more important homeopath in the world than Hans Wapler (1860-1951), editor of the *Allgemeinen Homoopathischen Zeitung,* whose publications were much neglected in America. Boyd set out to correct that by publishing Wapler's "The Incorporation of Homeopathy into United Medicine" in the *JAIH* in 1932. In it, Wapler took issue with those who condemned as traitors anyone who attempted to bridge the gulf between homeopathy and allopathy. "Our Hippocratic orientation in therapeutics has saved us from becoming sectarian," Wapler reasoned, preferring to be classified among those whose goal was not to set up similia in place of contraria but to have the homeopathic principle recognized as an "equally" regarded principle. Objecting to the goals of the Hahnemannians, he wrote: "We designate ourselves natural scientists since we place natural observation over speculation, over mental fabrication."[61]

Wapler criticized American homeopathy for its lack of scientific rigor. With the exception of the Wesselhoefts, he felt that few American physicians had worked for the scientific elaboration of homeopathy. This was also true of isopathy which had become so popular among orthodox Hahnemannians. With isopathy, "you have in your grasp, a wasp's nest," Wapler warned. He likewise questioned why Americans potentized beyond the thirtieth decimal. This remained "a puzzle for the ordinary mortal," he remarked. "We low potentists hold with [Johann Wolfgang von] Goethe that powerless material and material-less power are unauthorized abstractions." For Wapler there was not a "shadow of proof" that material-less specific drug powers actually existed.[62]

Taking steps to correct what he considered were fundamental weaknesses in homeopathy, John P. Sutherland, MD (b. 1854), professor of anatomy and dean of the Boston School of Medicine, recommended the establishment of research laboratories for the study of drug pathogenesy; a new materia medica that included only symptoms corroborated by repeated tests; the standardization of clinical reports; the teaching of courses on homeopathic theory, principles, and practice in the medical colleges; and continued support of homeopathic hospitals.[63] Homeopathy's progress had not been sufficient in the twentieth century because it had not developed a science upon which it could build a stable and enduring art. "No art can long survive without its necessary science" and, unfortunately, too many homeopaths were still using the drug provings handed down by Hahnemann and his immediate disciples. These were "so mixed with clinical symptoms and arranged in such an unimpressive and unattractive anatomical schema that the modern medical student is appalled, and turns hopelessly away." As a result, homeopathy was a house built on quicksand, unsupported by direct laboratory experimental evidence. Unless its foundations were strengthened with laboratory science and trained researchers, homeopathy would continue to face serious criticism from within and without.[64]

There was little question that the early followers of Hahnemann had set themselves apart from allopathy due to the latter's indiscriminate polypharmacy and overdosage, but the reasons behind this decision were no longer relevant, explained J. C. Hayner. "During the last thirty or forty years, a new aspect has been acquired which has tended strongly to eradicate the distinction between the two schools" he wrote. In point of fact, sectarianism and dogmatism had "largely ceased to exist."[65] Moreover, conditions had changed in the United States since the days when homeopathy had won wide support among the public. Newspapers no longer found it expedient to air differences among the schools, and allopathy's "open expression of antagonism" had all but disappeared. Added to this, the laity as a whole found it difficult to distinguish between the two schools since the application of the similia principle had become widely integrated into regular practice. "About all that is left to argue about resides in the interpretation of experimental data and the explanation of theories concerning the manner of drug selection and the degree of drug dosage," Hayner explained, "and the layman is not interested in experimentation and theory." This meant that the future of the homeopathic movement depended upon its appeal to members of the regular school. "It is no secret that there are many members of the old school who privately subscribe to the therapeutic principle for which we stand but who, because of their loyalty to their association, are unwilling to affirm their belief openly," he wrote. The future was clear. If ever homeopathy was to receive its due, it had to secure the "holy grail"—recognition as a specialty within regular medicine.[66]

The works of August Bier, Linn Boyd, William Boericke, Wilbert Hinsdale, Conrad Wesselhoeft, and Karl Kotschau made it easier for homeopaths to talk about homeopathy in terms of modern science and to offer objective laboratory proof of their theories. For Harold

R. Griffith, MD, Hahnemann had been a true scientist whose tools were his eyes, ears, and hands which he used with precision. "Had he lived one hundred years later he would have been adept in microscopy, and found value in the X-rays, the stethoscope and the electrocardiogram," he wrote. "He never intended us to believe that the last word in therapeutic progress had been enunciated with the *Organon*—his own constantly changing ideas prove that."[67]

LOOKING FOR SCAPEGOATS

Faced with the closing of their colleges and a precipitous decline in the status of homeopathy as a sect, it was not long before America's high-potency homeopaths began looking for scapegoats. Initially, several were identified—some obvious, others more obscure. Some blamed the abolition of the preceptor system which had been a time-honored custom with much to commend it. The influence of a good preceptor meant that students were "born to homeopathy" before entering medical school and carried their enthusiasm for homeopathic principles into their student days. Instead, students were now dissipating valuable time in fraternity life or worse, mimicking regular medicine. Others blamed state licensing boards that chose not to include examination in materia medica or therapeutics. A critic complained in 1922:

> Without preceptorial stimulus and with dozens of technical subjects to occupy his mind, most of which incidentally, [the medical student] will never need or use, small wonder that, unless his convictions regarding homeopathy are deep rooted, he will neglect the difficult study of homeopathic materia medica, especially when he knows that the state board . . . does not require it.

Still others concluded that they had made a fatal error in permitting state legislators to abolish separate examining boards. Homeopathic representation had been included on "unified" boards, but it had little practical value so far as the interests of homeopathy were concerned. To make matters worse, increasing numbers of homeopathic physicians acted "ashamed" of their professional identity and side-stepped the title whenever possible. No longer did doctors routinely place the designation of homeopath on their shingles, preferring instead to use the more generic title of doctor, MD, or physician.[68]

While the 1920s and 1930s served as the heyday of progressive homeopathy, the era also became a time of serious soul-searching. For Hahnemannians, too much energy had been spent on diagnostics and pathology at the expense of pharmacology and pharmaco-therapeutics. As a result, the unity of life, the unity of the human organism, and the unity of medicine had been sacrificed and, with them, a falling away of established methods, standards, and ideals. This criticism was lodged at some of homeopathy's most active university researchers who, in an effort to keep pace with regular medical colleges, were accused of wasting time doing work that was "useless and unworthy of their high standing and ability." Heedless to the concerns for homeopathy's future, they went about "uninstructed in the principles and methods of the sciences," and, lacking vision, perception, or historic perspective, endangered the very lifeblood of homeopathic philosophy. True homeopaths, remarked Hahnemannian Stuart M. Close, were hiding their faces in shame to see these "spoiled children" playing while their departments were closing down.[69]

In an article published in 1922 and titled "Sold Out," Alfred Pulford, MD (1863-1948), of Ohio warned that unless true believers were prepared to fight both the AIH and the AMA, homeopaths across the country would be compelled to swallow a bitter and humiliating pill. He accused the two organizations of "making love" to each other since the AIH underwent new leadership in 1919. As a result, "wooden-headed" homeopaths had become more or less "hypnotized" by the AMA and were even trying to remake the *JAIH* to "look like an appendix to the *JAMA*." Pulford accused Roy Upham, president of the AIH in 1921, of outright treason. "Perhaps Dr. Upham does not know which way he is going," complained Pulford. However, for all of Upham's upbeat comments, Pulford considered him a "Judas" within homeopathy and his actions little more than a "grandstand" effort that had all the earmarks of "pure unadulterated bluff." Believing that none but "true-blue" homeopaths should be admitted to the AIH, Pulford urged a thorough cleaning out of the national organization. As it presently stood, the organization was being led by "spineless jelly-fish" who were "dead from the neck up."[70]

Rudolph F. Rabe, president of the IHA in 1923, agreed with Pulford that the time spent on purely homeopathic subjects had been too curtailed in the remaining colleges. Homeopathy was no longer the central subject around which the curriculum was built. Instead of preparing "artists in homeopathic prescribing," the schools were producing graduates who could scarcely be distinguished from old school doctors.[71] For Rabe, homeopathy had suffered most from its friends by indulging in a "catholicity" of practice, namely, adopting a definition that defined a homeopathic physician in terms that constituted the "greatest latitude of practice." This expanded definition had been "diabolical in its Machiavellian cunning" by granting to the homeopathic physician a license to "indulge in veritable orgies of kaleidoscopic therapeutic heterodoxy." This was tragically wrong. Insofar as homeopathy intended to retain its sectarian character, it was essential for the homeopathic physician to practice homeopathy and nothing else. This meant practicing therapeutics on the basis of the Law of Similia, employing minimum doses, one remedy at a time. Short of that, homeopathy's institutions would quietly disappear, and probably should, shorn of their ability to practice genuine homeopathy. He blamed the AIH for being "neglectful of the basic interests of the science and art of homeopathy."[72]

In reflecting on his own earlier medical training at Hahnemann in Philadelphia, Donald A. Davis of Pittsburgh remarked that less than 5 percent of his class knew anything more than "like cures like" and the names of a few of the remedies in the homeopathic materia medica. "In our most famous homeopathic college in the United States, there is comparatively little chance for a man to become acquainted with the desirable methods of practicing homeopathic medicine," he stated. More to the point, many of Hahnemann's basic teachings were "openly opposed" by the faculty at the college. Like others of his generation, Davis believed that homeopathy would have been far better off taught as a specialty.[73]

STUART M. CLOSE

The face of homeopathy was seriously disquieted when Stuart M. Close (1860-1929), founder of the Brooklyn Hahnemannian Union in 1896, teacher at the New York Homeopathic Medical College from

1909 to 1913, and editor of the Department of Homeopathic Philosophy for the *Homeopathic Recorder,* observed that homeopathy had "simply stood, marking time," carrying the legacies bequeathed by its ancestors. Its pharmacology and therapeutics had not been extended or improved and the standards of practice set by Hahnemann were being kept alive by only a few true believers. Although there had been some research illustrative of the Law of Similia, little had been done to establish Hahnemann's corollary principles. In looking at the state of homeopathy in America, Close conceded that most college graduates had drifted far from Hahnemann's teachings and, like their allopathic brethren, had become "empirical generalizers and routinists." Since the *Organon,* the *Materia Medica Pura,* and the *Chronic Diseases* were no longer studied, Hahnemann's beliefs and practices were rapidly going out of existence. Whether they disappeared or were regenerated into something new and better remained a question. Just as everything in nature was continually dying and being reborn, Close hoped that homeopathy would be part of that universal and cosmic rhythm of life.[74] The soul of homeopathy was not dead, "but waiting, like the daughter of Jarius for the Master to come, and say, 'Weep not; she is not dead, but sleepeth.'"[75]

As the official ideologue of the IHA's Bureau of Homeopathic Philosophy, Close represented and advocated on behalf of those therapeutic specialists who "stood for the development and maintenance of the distinctive principles and methods of homeopathy as it was given to the world by Hahnemann." In his view, the bureau's purpose was to "redeem homeopathy from the many corruptions and perversions which had crept into its practice." Close had been a student of Bernhardt Fincke and Phineas Parkhurst Wells and, like them, advocated pure Hahnemannianism. In 1906, he was elected president of the IHA and represented the heart and soul of Hahnemannianism in the post–World War I era.[76] Under Close's guidance, the Bureau of Homeopathic Philosophy became the subject of criticism in that what it advanced as science was also a philosophy closely bound to the ideas of a single individual. For Close, this was no impediment any more than Jesus was for Christianity, Newton for the law of gravitation, or the authors Matthew, Mark, Luke, and John for the Bible. Homeopathic philosophy was like any other branch of philosophy in that it dealt with general principles, laws, and theories. The source of its philosophy was the *Organon,* and its originator and founder was Hahnemann. Close felt that, like the Bible, the *Organon* could be read and understood by anyone of average intelligence, including laypersons, but required scholars and specialists in the history of philosophy and science to plumb its more erudite citations and allusions, its nomenclature, and its dogmatic tone. For Close, homeopathy was "a sane, pure, rational philosophy, with a definite, scientific, therapeutic method and a highly developed practical technique, all systematized and based upon a universal principle or law of nature."[77]

Close explained the reformer's lot as one of turbulence, self-sacrifice, struggle, and danger. Such had been the case with Copernicus and Galileo, with John Wycliffe and Johannes Huss, with Martin Luther and Ulrich Zwingli, and so too with Hahnemann. All were "protestants." According to Close,

> homeopathy is the original protestant offshoot from the "Romish Church"' of medicine, and Hahnemann was its Luther. It represents the revolt of thinking, progressive men against the tyranny of tradition; against corrupt alliances and perversion of principles, against ignorance, bigotry and intolerance; against medical "priestcraft" and aggression; against "Medical Trusts" and oligarchies, all of which have had and still have representation and embodiment in medicine.[78]

Admitting that Hahnemann's teachings were difficult to explain in the language of modern bacteriology, Close nonetheless felt that scholars could easily discover in what manner the psora theory had anticipated the later discoveries of Robert Koch (1843-1910) and Louis Pasteur (1822-1895). Unfortunately, the medical world had become so "obsessed" with bacteriology that it had "lost sight of the individual altogether," forcing therapeutic applications on patients that were "neither legitimate nor scientific." True, bacteriology was a factor in disease, but there were too many other elements that needed to be taken into consideration. "Not to recognize these facts is to open the way to grave abuses and misapplications," warned Close. Thus, the current wave of serums, vaccines, and antitoxins and their administration via the hypodermic needle was "productive of incalculable injury." Under the sway of bacteriology, the key elements of clinical history and symptomatology had become a "lost art." In their place, orthodox medicine had introduced serum and vaccine treatment as the *sine qua non* for cure.[79]

In an address before the American Foundation for Homeopathy in 1925, Close explained that homeopathy as a school and as an institution was facing a critical moment. Not only were its colleges going out of existence, but older practitioners were also dying off faster than they could be replaced. In addition, its hospitals had passed into the hands of regulars or were under the control of individuals who were only nominally homeopathic. The same was true of its once vibrant societies. Few were still functioning. As for the majority of the rank and file, it was difficult to speak of them "without indignation and grief." Ignorant of homeopathy's history, its theories and its principles, and perceived as accepting every new product of modern scientific medicine, licensed practitioners were no longer viewed as spokesmen for true homeopathy. Instead, they had become the product of "four generations of degenerating ancestors, each worse than the last."[80]

Nonetheless, all was not lost. Noting that a cadre of loyal homeopaths had held to the highest standards of practice (i.e., Clemens Boenninghausen, Johann E. Staph, Gustav W. Gross, Constantine Hering, Adolph Lippe, Henry N. Guernsey, William Wesselhoeft, Carroll Dunham, Phineas P. Wells, Benjamin F. Joslin, Bernhardt Fincke, James Tyler Kent, and Henry C. Allen), Close explained that it was now necessary to separate the methods and principles of homeopathy from its institutions in the same manner that it had once been necessary to separate Christianity from the Catholic Church. Organizations were always dying, but truth continually re-embodied itself in new forms of organization. "It is always alive, always active, always in transition," he jubilantly explained. Rather than be discouraged, he urged his audience to appreciate the broader extent of the changes going on and the part they were playing in the new educational enterprise.[81]

THINKING THE INEVITABLE

In 1935, the Council on Medical Education and Hospitals of the AMA gave notice that after July 1, 1938, it would "no longer carry on its approved list schools of sectarian medicine." In response to the resolution, the board of trustees of the AIH on November 21, 1935, resolved to maintain a united front to the public while preparing itself to meet with AMA representatives to work out an amicable solution provided that they could continue to call their institutions homeopathic. The organization was prepared to take their case to the courts and to the public should the AMA persist in denying homeopaths the right to name their own institutions and to teach their own therapeutics. Similar resolutions were passed by the Eastern Homeopathic Medical Association, various Ohio associations, the Connecticut Homeopathic Medical Society, and the Allegheny County Homeopathic Medical Society. Representatives of the Huron Road Hospital Staff, Cleveland-Pulte Homeopathic Medical College, the Ohio State Homeopathic Medical Society, and the Cleveland Homeopathic Medical Society passed resolutions calling upon the two remaining colleges "to stay all action in regards to the demands of the Council of Medical Education of the AMA until cooperative action of the homeopathic forces can bring its strength into action."[82]

Prior to the decisions taken by the New York Homeopathic Medical College and Flower Hospital and by the Hahnemann Medical College of Philadelphia there were debates by members of the two faculties; signed statements of preferences given by alumni; and discussions with their respective trustees and with the AIH. However, as was stated in an editorial in the *JAIH,* the matter ultimately rested with the trustees of the two institutions.[83]

In 1936, Dean Claude A. Burrett, MD of the New York Homeopathic Medical College and Flower Hospital, met with members of the AIH to review the past history of the school, its recent progress, the publications of its faculty, and his decision to change its name to the New York Medical College and Flower Hospital. Burrett explained that the action taken by the AMA's Council on Medical Education made it impossible for any college with other than a class "A" rating to secure students and to assure that its graduates obtained internships and licenses to practice. Burrett expressed the opinion that the dropping of the name, which implied sectarianism, would place the institution "in a position such that it would be able to obtain the best teachers . . . without restricting the teaching of homeopathy."[84] The college would reserve sixteen hourly sessions for homeopathy, with formal lectures and the formation of proving groups. Students could elect to study homeopathy more thoroughly if they chose; otherwise, they could choose surgery or one of the other specialties. "All we can do now is to give the students a broad vision of Homeopathy and a clear understanding of its basic principles; the rest is on the laps of the gods," reported doctors E. Wallace MacAdam and William Gutman.[85] By contrast, Hahnemann Medical College of Philadelphia announced that it had no intention of ending instruction in homeopathy or changing its name.[86] It retained an elective course on the program inventory as well as a postgraduate "Doctorate in Homeopathic Therapeutics."

Although homeopaths looked with pride at the towering structure that was Hahnemann Hospital on North Broad Street in Philadelphia and admired the beautiful Fifth Avenue Hospital in New York City, they could not help but feel that the last several years had been devastating to their cause. First had been the order to curtail the number of hours devoted to the teaching of homeopathic therapeutics in their curricula. Next was the order to remove the word "homeopathic" from the official name. Finally came the suggestion that as vacancies arose on their respective faculties, they were to be filled with men and women from the old school rather than from homeopathy. In view of these changes, the vulnerability of homeopathy's future was most certainly evident.[87]

By the late 1940s, it was still possible to find optional or elective lectures on homeotherapeutics in the undergraduate curriculum of three medical colleges. The New York Medical College assigned thirty hours to the subject over its four-year program. Its teacher was Dr. E. W. MacAdam. In Philadelphia, Hahnemann Medical College assigned seventy hours to the subject over a four-year period. The instructor of record, Dr. Garth W. Boericke (1893-1968), taught the principles of homeopathy and the materia medica. On the Pacific coast, the University of California at Berkeley maintained a chair in homeopathy but only about 10 percent of the students elected to take a course in the subject.[88]

ON REFLECTION

The rush to establish medical colleges in nineteenth century America was a phenomenon common to all of the leading medical systems—regular, homeopathic, eclectic, and physio-medical. By the end of the nineteenth century, 162 schools of all grades and types were operating. Similarly, the closing of schools in the twentieth century became a national phenomenon as well. By 1937, only seventy-seven Class "A" schools remained in existence.[89] In towns and cities across the United States where homeopathic physicians had once practiced, homeopathy had become little more than a distant memory. Without colleges or hospitals, and with the passing of the older generation of doctors, homeopathy was relegated to an "almost forgotten and outmoded cult beyond the realm of serious consideration." Even in those schools where homeopathy lingered as a "voluntary" course, few students expressed sufficient interest to enroll.[90]

By the end of the Second World War, the graduates of homeopathy's last remaining colleges who had served in the armed forces had learned the importance of antibiotics and were more than willing to accept the products of modern medicine. While homeopathy was seemingly in its death throes, and as the AIH continued to lose membership and influence, IHA members began extending their influence into the AIH to undertake its regeneration. These hard-line believers were not so much interested in opening the field to the laity as much as remedying the professional side of homeopathy with more philosophically based medicine. Indeed, argued Julian Winston, the literature was so "full of vitality" that while the IHA had only 147 members in 1944, it nonetheless pulsated with a sense of its power. Thus, while progressive homeopaths had embarked on intensive efforts to transform their colleges according to Flexnerian standards, or close them if they failed to make the grade, conservatives argued that this emulation of regular medical education standards violated the very intentions behind their establishment and, feeling few regrets, moved toward an alternative system of postgraduate education. Despite the refusal of the AMA to recognize homeopathy as a specialty, the Diplomate of Homeotherapeutics stood as a visible sign of homeopathy's stalwart allegiance to classical homeopathy and apart from both the older pseudo-homeopathy and the newer winds of lay homeopathy.[91]

In assessing modern American homeopathy, the significance of its failed colleges can scarcely be overstated. What emerged from their slow demise before the political, economic, social, and cultural dominance of conventional medicine was a sense of betrayal, still felt today, against homeopathy's early leaders who chose to invest their precious resources in bricks and mortar rather than in postgraduate education or in chairs of medicine. One can hypothesize what homeopathy may have become had it avoided replicating the educational system of conventional medicine. Would its relationship with conventional medicine have been any different? Would it have obtained its "holy grail" of being recognized as a specialty within conventional medicine? Would homeopathy have chosen a road other than the high dilutions? Would medically educated homeopaths have allowed laypersons to compete with their own claims of legitimacy? Would homeopathy be more science- than faith-based?

From what we know regarding homeopath's history, some would argue that had homeopathy become a specialty within conventional medicine, there would have been more "science" than "belief" in its practices; greater skepticism as to the primacy of Hahnemann's literal teachings; a scaling down of the higher dilutions; greater research using the double-blind controlled clinical trials; a diminution of the role of laypersons in the caregiving process; the continuance of homeopathic practices within the medical paradigm; and the maintenance of tighter licensing standards. Above all, there would have been fewer fads and heretical perspectives, and a marked reduction in the intensity of disputes between and among homeopathy's well-organized and influential interest groups. No doubt some controversy would continue to live on in small pockets but the proto-orthodoxy of low-potency homeopathy would probably have prevailed and been tolerated by conventional medicine.

Chapter 2

Esoteric Homeopathy

While academic homeopathy died at the hands of both conservative and progressive homeopaths—each for different reasons—classical, esoteric, or Hahnemannian homeopathy continued its journey into the twentieth century. Among proponents, classical homeopathy implied allegiance to an original and unwavering set of correct principles. It seems clear, however, that aside from an adherence to the theory of vitalism, few principles remained intact for very long. Instead one finds any number of individuals purporting to connect fragments of Samuel Hahnemann's writings with their own ideological proclivities. Out of this emerged many competing and often divergent practices, each seeking a kind of historical validation in which old and new ideas were melded into a plausible synthesis. All claimed authenticity and all competed in the marketplace of ideas as the true art and science of homeopathy. In this sense, we can say that there have been multiple homeopathies, each claiming title to correct belief. Reviewed in this chapter are several variations that, at one time or another, purported to represent the authentic corpus of homeopathic thought. That they succeeded in winning the hearts and minds of so many is testament to their appeal and creativity. That they were also capable of claiming support within the conservative wing of homeopathy suggests the need for rethinking what classical or Hahnemannian homeopathy really meant to this system of reform medicine.[1]

VITALISM

Along with a number of competing alternative and complementary medical systems in the nineteenth and twentieth centuries, homeopathy affirmed the existence of a "vital force" or "vital energy" that pervaded the universe and which could be drawn upon to activate, provoke, redirect, or protect a diseased or disordered organism. This force or energy was more than just physical or mechanical in nature; rather it was a "spiritual," "universal intelligence," "psychic," "innate," or "auric" power which in past times had variously been called the "vis medicatrix naturae," "anima," "sensitive soul," "principe vitale," or "vital principle." It was a power unbounded by the laws of physics.[2] For the esoteric wing of homeopathy, life represented an immaterial, independent, and dynamic force that presided over and moved the organic structure. It was the power through which the organism performed its functions; it was not the sum of the functions, but their "moving cause." Health represented a state in which the entities of matter (chemical), spirit (human sympathies), and life (vitalism) acted in a normal and balanced manner. In disease, however, morbid elements entered the organism and manifested themselves in symptoms, the outward signs of the body's imbalance. These morbid elements could lie dormant for weeks, months, even years, with little or no outward manifestations. In most instances, they were met and expelled by the organism's own powers (*vis medicatrix naturae*), but on other occasions, more substantive energies were required to assist in the body's repair.[3]

Just as each individual had a particular personality or constitution, so also did drugs such as aconite, belladonna, silex, sulphur, nux vomica, and pulsatilla. While nature had within it the capacity to cure disease, with or without the assistance of external stimulants, disease was hurried or retarded by such stimuli as the homeopathist could bring to bear on the powers of nature. For example, when the personality of a specific drug was brought in contact with the personality of an individual person, according to the Law of Similia, a corrective balance was assured. However small the drug atom, it could produce symptoms of a certain character. Even when the external molecule was so small that it no longer remained in the solution, there were those who believed an "imprint" of the drug remained behind to cling to the medium and thus affect the body in some fashion. Thus, while less general laws worked their cure in certain situations, the only permanent cure occurred when the morbid influence was "neutralized" by Hahnemann's potentized materia medica.[4]

Given that homeopaths viewed disease as entering the body through one of three portals—molecular, spiritual, or vital affinities—it followed that remedies could be introduced in the same manner. They could be digested and absorbed through the material side; enter on the spiritual side in the form of thoughts and emotions; or through life itself by way of the vital character. When disease came by way of the material side, the patient's constitution (personality) was treated by changing the condition of the body itself with the introduction of specific drug molecules. Thus, when molecules of metallic arsenic were absorbed by the living organism, they became part of the patient's personality as they moved through the body and were deposited throughout the system. If the remedial approach came by way of the passions and emotions, the intellectual operations of the body were modified through mental impressions. Finally, if the remedial approach was through the vital essence (i.e., life itself), it was accomplished through the spiritual sphere by these influences alone.[5]

A "vital" remedy was one whose energy detached from its natural material source and relocated into an artificial medium (i.e., sugar of milk) and from which it was appropriated by the vital force or spirit of the patient. Most of the valuable remedial agents were substances that, until potentized, were wholly inert. When potentized, explained Rufus Choate in 1888, their spirit-like medicinal powers were "invisible, imponderable, and will never be discerned by the most powerful microscope or the closest chemical analysis." The first dose of an appropriate dynamic medicine was intended to produce on the system results corresponding to the impressions produced by the disease. If the dose was similar in kind and of sufficient potency, it brought the vital force to the point of overthrowing the disease. If the dose was not similar, or was contrary, a counter force caused a reaction and the disease reappeared in a more aggressive manner.[6] This was the "crowning glory of our system," reasoned homeopath Roger G. Perkins, and was as much a revelation to the practice of medicine as the Christian religion had been to mankind. The homeopathic proposition that the ultimate atom contained specific qualities that were intensified by friction had become an article of the homeopath's "medical creed."[7]

While American and some English homeopaths felt at home in the metaphysical world of vitalism and the higher potencies, their German counterparts were less inclined to follow the same muse. In his *Lehrbuch der Homeopathie,* Eduard von Grauvogl (1811-1877) sought to counter the mental and spiritual notions held by homeopathy's "transcendental" supporters and replace them with a more materialistic view of medical science. Grauvogl followed in the footsteps of the great naturalist Charles Darwin (1809-1882), English philosopher Herbert Spencer (1820-1903), and German biologist and philosopher Ernst Haeckel (1834-1919) in believing that the world of matter worked well without necessitating a corresponding world of spiritual agencies. The chemical and physical laws alone were sufficient to account for the manifestations of nature. In saying this, Grauvogl repudiated the doctrine of vital force; opposed the belief that remedies acted dynamically by virtue of an inherent power; and defended the use of multiple drugs. He argued that the Law of Similia was limited by certain boundaries and did not supersede the principle of contraries; rather, the two principles "reciprocally complete each other."[8]

American homeopaths of the Hahnemannian persuasion rejected Grauvogl's materialism, preferring to believe in the existence of a more mysterious power or spirit acting upon the tissues of the organism. Physical stimuli were not enough to originate life and the material organism was itself not a living machine. When Hahnemann moved his system of homeopathy in the direction of dynamism, vital force became the indwelling ruler of the physical organism, or what James Tyler Kent called the "viceregent."[9] With this new principle that Hahnemann introduced into pharmacology, he also developed simultaneously a new pathology and a new therapeutics.

Another popular proponent of vitalism at the turn of the twentieth century was Hans Driesch (1867-1941) of the University of Heidelberg whose Gifford lectures given at the University of Aberdeen were later published in the *Science and Philosophy of the Organism* (1908). In these lectures, Driesch located the life principle in the protoplasm. This was unlike the older vitalism of Plato, Paracelsus, and Georg Ernst Stahl who viewed the vital principle as distinct from chemical and other physical forces. Driesch, on the other hand, relied on the Aristotelian hypothesis of *entelechy* to explain the relationship of the immaterial entity within the organism. Later in his *History and Theory of Vitalism* (1914), Dreisch traced the evolution of vitalism from the theories of Aristotle, Harvey, and Stahl, through the writings of Gustav Wolff, William Roux, C. Lloyd Morgan, Albrecht von Haller, John F. Blumenbach, Immanuel Kant, Justus von Liebig and Arthur Schopenhauer, Henri Bergson, to others in more modern times. The terms "vitalism," "neovitalism," "dynamis," "dynamism," "vital force," "vital energy," "sensorium," and "potentiality" were terms commonly used by Dreisch and the neovitalists of the 1920s and were strikingly similar to the language of Hahnemann and his more metaphysical advocates. According to Benjamin C. Woodbury of Massachusetts, homeopathy, vitalism, and neovitalism were all attributes of true Hahnemannianism.[10]

EMANUEL SWEDENBORG

Contemporaneous with Hahnemann's journey from low- to high-potency medicine and the advocacy of a vital energy that acted upon the organism, American homeopaths were supported by the spiritual and scientific writings of Swedish scientist, philosopher, and religious writer Emanuel Swedenborg (1666-1772) whose books were translated from Latin into English by Dr. Garth Wilkinson (1812-1899). Wilkinson also wrote a biography of Swedenborg, published in 1849. It was through Henry James, Sr., editor of *The Harbinger* of New York, a Fourierist newspaper, that Wilkinson was introduced to homeopathy and underwent a gradual conversion to Hahnemann's principles. In doing so, Wilkinson introduced into homeopathy the spiritual and esoteric ideas of Swedenborg, contributing an altogether new understanding to the modus operandi of Hahnemann's high dilutions. Wilkinson was convinced that Swedenborg's law of correspondences (i.e., individuals have a living relationship with the visible and invisible world surrounding them thus allowing individuals to see the causes behind actions which are usually taken for granted) could explain the virtues of *similia similibus curantur,* drug and disease effects, the connection between the physical and the psychological, and the bridge between the soul, brain, and body. He furthermore believed that the law of correspondences provided a teleological or purposive notion for a universe whose formative elements—finites, actives, magnetic, and etheric—were both visible and invisible. Just as "New Church" Swedenborgians viewed the world as a gradual descent from the spiritual through a series of degrees to the visible and physical universe, the so-called New School homeopaths recognized disease as having a spiritual causation manifesting itself in a symptom-complex on the material body. Indeed, the nineteenth-century cults of transcendentalism, Swedenborgianism,

Mesmerism, Fourierism, animal magnetism, and sarcognomy were all in some manner connected to the concept of vitality and its influence over the various organs and functions of the human body.[11]

Author, translator, and critic Charles Julius Hempel (1811-1879), chair of materia medica and therapeutics at the Hahnemann Medical College of Philadelphia, tried to find a middle ground between the hard and fast beliefs of the materialists and the high-potency wing of homeopathy. For him, vitalism was "the very corner stone" of Hahnemann's therapeutics and therefore he considered it impossible to give an intelligible account of the Law of Similia and the operation of small doses without inferring something beyond a strict materialism. An admirer of Swedenborg, Hempel thought that the law of correspondences and theories of influx and degrees bore a more appropriate relationship to the fundamental principles of homeopathy. "The day is fast approaching," Hempel predicted, "when the homeopathic profession will bow to Swedenborg as the great expounder of the philosophy of homeopathy." For the present, however, far too much importance had been attached to the so-called high potencies as a "badge of a superior Homeopathy." These were "ridiculous pretensions" that had no place in the true science of homeopathy. Although he did not deny outright the powers in the higher potencies, at least in the abstract, they could not be realized without "the intercession of their natural substratum in the world of matter."[12] Hempel's effort to establish a "medium school" of homeopathic medicine was harshly repudiated by the school's conservative wing which viewed vitalism, potentization of drugs, the Law of Similia, drug provings, and individualization of remedy and patient as the school's most distinctive attributes.[13]

In 1888, the *Homeopathic Recorder* reviewed Emanuel Swedenborg's *The Soul: Or Rational Psychology* (1887), translated by Frank Sewell and published in New York by the New Church Board of Publication. Although it was unusual for a medical journal to review a book professedly dealing with theology, the editors justified the review by pointing out that as a thinker and philosopher, Swedenborg had made an enduring impression on the age. The distinctions of soul, mind, and animus brought out in his writings, as well as his use of the terms "ether," "spiral," "vortical motion," "subtile spirit," and what he called the "nervous fluid," had made him a contributor to some of the great questions in science.[14] Swedenborg believed that everything existed within three discrete degrees: a soul degree, or the inmost; an intermediate degree; and an ultimate or outmost degree. The three degrees were distinct planes of activity with the higher degrees acting upon the lower ones. For homeopaths who read his works, the planes seemed to support in descending order the soul, the vital force, and the material body.[15]

Notwithstanding the efforts of Hempel and others to connect homeopathy with Swedenborgianism, it remained for James Tyler Kent (1849-1916) to entice several generations of American homeopaths into a more formalized association with Swedenborgianism.[16] A native of New York, Kent was educated in medicine at the Eclectic Medical Institute of Cincinnati, graduating in 1871. He began his medical career as an eclectic but turned his attention to homeopathy following an illness which befell his second wife and failed to yield to either eclectic or allopathic treatment. He became a student of Hahnemann's *Organon,* resigned from the Eclectic Medical Association in 1879, and took a teaching appointment in the Homeopathic Medical College of Missouri from 1881 to 1888. He later became dean and professor of materia medica in the Post Graduate School of Homeopathics in Philadelphia, dean and professor of materia medica in Dunham Medical College of Chicago, dean and professor of materia medica in Hering Medical College of Chicago, and also in Hahnemann Medical College of Chicago.

It is difficult to understand Kent's views on high dilutions without recognizing how immensely Swedenborg's beliefs contributed to the formulation of his hierarchy of symptoms "from innermost to the outermost," and his degrees of potencies.[17] Kent's combination of Hahnemannian and Swedenborgian thought became the centerpiece for high dilutionists and a real dividing line between materialists looking to physio-chemical changes and vitalists intent on discovering degrees of matter and spirit in their substances. Kent's philosophy was double-edged. While it provided an underpinning for homeopathic doctrines in America and in some Western European countries, it carried with it the attributes of religious belief and a style which historian Peter Morrell characterized as "akin to that of a fundamentalist preacher," thus making it less relevant to more progressive homeopaths.[18] Kent effectively moved homeopathy away from the more eclectic and experimental medicine of the late nineteenth century with its emphasis on scientific rationalism, to a more metaphysical and dogmatic approach that connected man's "innermost spiritual to his outermost natural."[19] Kent focused on the strict application of Hahnemann's basic laws: the Law of Similia, the single remedy, and the minimum dose. Added to these applications were his hierarchy of symptoms and a repertory based on Swedenborg's notions of body, mind, and soul. As Kentianism became synonymous with Swedenborgianism, progressive homeopaths found themselves dragged further and further away from the rigors of modern science and laboratory-based medicine.

Swedenborg's influence was later recognized by Dean John P. Sutherland in his address at the opening exercises of the forty-seventh annual session of the Boston University School of Medicine in October 1919. He remarked that two main philosophies within homeopathy had squared off against each other. The one, represented in the writings of German biologist and philosopher Ernst Haeckel stood for materialism guided by science. Haeckel's religion was "Monism," a term he invented to cover his belief in the essential unity of organic and inorganic matter. The other was set by Swedenborg who welcomed the teachings of science and gladly accepted Revelation along with it.[20] While Sutherland found himself among the progressive set of homeopaths who had aligned themselves with the empirically based system of science and medicine, others found the siren calls of the Swedenborgians more appealing. A belief in an "immaterial something" that dwelt with the living being had been found in the writings of many of the ancient peoples and their scholars, explained Charles L. Olds, but it was not until Swedenborg that a new and rational theory of the vital principle was given to the world of science and philosophy. Without his philosophy, homeopaths were "left in the dark as to a rational explanation of . . . homeopathic law and principles." For Olds, the esoteric aspects of Hahnemann's medicine could only be understood within the context of the doctrines contained in Swedenborg's philosophy.[21]

HOMEOPATHY AS A BELIEF SYSTEM

When the president of the AIH addressed delegates in 1889 with the words "believers in the law of similars," the editor of *Medical Advance* complained that homeopathicians were tired of the words "faith" and "belief" in the practice of their science. Faith was not the principle upon which homeopathy was founded; rather, it was knowledge of what a remedy could do through its provings.[22] Despite this correction, homeopathy had indeed become a belief system in the United States, triggered by emphasis on high-potency medicines, Swedenborgianism, and the overarching dominance of Kentian ideas that all but suppressed the low-potency progressive elements among academically trained homeopaths. For Stuart M. Close of the *Homeopathic Recorder,* homeopathy was founded on the "bed-rock of a belief in and recognition of the Living God" as explained by Hahnemann in his doctrine of the "Life Force." This belief connected Hahnemann with the great schools of philosophic and religious thought and separated homeopathy from the materialistic philosophies of more modern times that had replaced God with a blind and unintelligent "energy" or "force."[23]

According to Benjamin C. Woodbury (1882-1948) who taught the principles of homeopathy at the Boston University School of Medicine and later served as president of the IHA, the medical world was in desperate need of a restatement of faith in the healing power of nature. In the mind of every follower of Hahnemann, this power had been the strongest element in the healing process. It was, in fact, this element upon which "the very character of the true Hahnemannian depends." Not only had it stood against regular medicine's failure to progress much "beyond the pale of superstition, dogmatism, and medievalism," it also held ground against the host of drugless cults "adrift in hopeless confusion upon the great sea of psychological and metaphysical formulas." Both extremes, he felt, were in need of guidance. Homoeopathy, alone among the schools of medicine, provided such a guide—the Law of Similia.[24]

For Woodbury, Hahnemann remained the preeminent medical philosopher, formulating in clear and unmistakable language the theory of vitalism. Moreover, his doctrines of attenuation and potentization presaged the discovery of radium and electron theory which would, Woodbury predicted, ultimately vindicate the followers of Hahnemann by opening a new "dogmatic atomistic era" in homoeopathy. For the future, he urged homeopaths to look at the universe as being in "a constant state of vibratory activity," in a struggle between positive and negative forces, where Swedenborg's law of correspondences provided a more complete understanding of the intricate subtleties that connected every phenomenon. Woodbury thought, too, that the discovery of radium confirmed the basic principles of the homeopathic law of potency, showing that even molecules beyond the third centesimal trituration were in stages of vigorous motion.[25]

For classical homeopaths, Hahnemann had "beat the modern scientists to their goals." By this Alfred Pulford meant that science had reached the molecule, the atom, and the ion and had now arrived at the electron. All this had been presaged by Hahnemann who "sensed what lay beyond the electron when he advised potentizing . . . remedies." Kent carried it even further when he urged taking remedies "on up the scale." Recognizing that disease had its origin in the "ultra-microscopical cells," homeopaths concluded that the only effective way to influence them was to approach them with the same ultra-microscopical medicines. Sera, toxins, vaccines, and low-potencies drugs were failures because of their crudity. Cures attributed to them were short-lived, returning after a temporary suppression or diversion.[26]

Others were similarly inclined to define homeopathy as representing some level of metaphysical existence. For example, Stuart Close classified the various schools of philosophy as *materialistic, idealistic* (or spiritualistic), and *substantialistic.* The materialist theories, of which there were many, regarded all species of sentient and mental life as products of the organism, and the universe as the product of physical elements. By contrast, idealists viewed the universe as the realization of a system of ideas. The third school, what Close called substantialism, held that all things in nature—whether principles, forces of nature, or the atoms of corporeal bodies—were really substantial entities that included the life and mental powers of every sentient organism. In other words, the mind was as real in its existence as the physical brain. This theory, proposed by A. Wilford Hall in his *The Problem of Human Life,* published in 1877, meant that gravity, magnetism, sound, light, heat, and electricity were substantial emanations. Within every living creature there existed a vital and mental organism, an invisible counterpart of its physical structure. Close thought that Hahnemann and his disciples fit the substantialist classification better than the idealist or spiritualist categories.[27]

As Close explained, Hahnemann conceptualized two versions of vital force. The first was an "unreasoning life-force" or principle that was unintelligent, blind, crude, and untrustworthy in health. This vital force was not guided by reason, knowledge, or reflection, but acted according to the physical constitution of the organism. However, the life or mind, in a cosmic sense, was much more than that. "Life in the individual being is the sum total of all the elementary organic forces, derived from and inseparably united with the universal or cosmic life, or being," Close wrote. "In the individual, life is a continuous influx from the life of the Universal and Infinite Being, and finds its perfect manifestation through organism, in spiritual and physical harmony or health." Said another way, the mind of each human being was connected with the cosmic whole and therefore an organ within a larger living organism.[28]

Using this latter metaphor, it was easy for Hahnemannians to reject allopathy as "circumscribed in its blind materialism, limited by the analytical researches of the laboratory [and] drowned in the multiplicity of diagnostic detail." Allopathy concentrated its attention on the organ, ignoring the body as a whole. It treated the physical "without regard to the spiritual, without knowing the mind, without concern for the differences of temperament and character except recently along the broadest lines, thus only knowing the negative portion of its domain: illness and death." Acute diseases were simply "warded off by vaccines, or choked by strong drugs." And when they modulated into "persistent humoral taints and in glandular devitalization," they degenerated into chronic affections. Unlike allopathy, the school of homeopathy did not camouflage symptoms. It attacked chronic diseases "plane by plane" and cured the patient "soundly and irreversibly" through spiritual and physical "purification." Looking at the matter philosophically, Dr. Pierre Schmidt (1894-1987) of Geneva, Switzerland, who was responsible for reintroducing classical homeopathy into Europe, envisaged medicine as bordering on philosophy and the doctor as "a synthetic savant and a spiritual initiate, welded into one." In treating patients with a few globules of drug on the tongue, the homeopathic physician not only knew the value and scope of his remedies, but also had the responsibility for educating his patient "to make him understand the necessity of aligning himself with the sacred mandates of the law." The physician gave his patients lessons in "biologic philosophy," a task substantively different from the materialistic allopathic physician.[29]

HIGH POTENCIES

Writing in 1890, Dr. Robert E. Dudgeon (1820-1904), an advocate of low-potency medicines, noted that there was a "noisy, if not very numerous" group within homeopathy who had arrogated to themselves the title of Hahnemannians and published their cases under the rubric of "Hahnemannian Homeopathy" and "Hahnemannian Cures." Given the presumptuous claims made by these self-styled purists, Dudgeon thought it time to set forth Hahnemann's true mode of practice from those who seemed particularly bent on casting aspersions on any practices not following their own interpretation of the master. Using the 1833 edition of Hahnemann's *Materia Medica,* Dudgeon pointed out that the author had directed practitioners to select only those medicines whose effects on the healthy body corresponded to the totality of the symptoms of the disease. This admonition also appeared in Hahnemann's *Organon* and in his *Chronic Diseases.* Hahnemann, he argued, was similarly emphatic as to the need for practitioners to prepare their medicines in the same manner and described in great detail how this was to be accomplished. Some medicines were to be diluted with spirits of wine through thirty different phials up to the 30th potency, and activated with a specific number of shakes. Others were to be triturated with milk sugar and further attenuated with spirits of wine through twenty-seven phials. But "how widely the self-styled Hahnemannists have departed from Hahnemann's instructions!" exclaimed Dudgeon. Hahnemann's reason for selecting the 30th potency as the standard dose for general use was due to his repeated admonition: "I do not approve of your dynamizing the medicines higher—as, for instance, up to 36 and 60. There must be some end to the thing; it cannot go on to infinity." Increasing the number of dilutions beyond the 30th potency, reasoned Dudgeon, had caused critics to reproach homeopaths with having no fixed or normal standard. True, Hahnemann did not condemn Russian homeopath Iseman von Korsakoff (d. 1853) for his extreme potencies but he advised followers not to go beyond the 30th dilution. In the last edition of the *Organon,* he alluded to dilutions as high as 300 but did not recommend them. Thus, if a physician commenced with the 30th dilution, he should next give a 24th, then an 18th, next the 12th, and finally the 6th. In other words, succeeding doses, if given, should be administered in lower, not higher dilutions.[30]

By contrast, Hahnemannians preferred attenuations at the 200th, and more frequently at the 1,000th, 10,000th, or even millionth—preparations designated on the authority of manufacturers like German Julius Caspar Jenichen (1787-1849), Samuel Swan (1814-1893), Bernhardt Fincke (1821-1906), Thomas Skinner (1825-1906), Ellis M. Santee, Ehrhart and Karl, and Boericke and Tafel, each with his own distinctive method of preparation. Fincke, a graduate of New York University School of Medicine and president of the IHA in 1896, claimed that no dose was ever too small. His remedies were manufactured in potencies as high as 40,000.[31]

Not only were these dilutions in total disregard for Hahnemann's wishes, complained Dudgeon, but the experience of a practitioner using Jenichen's potentizer was substantively different from one who used Fincke's, Swans's, Foote's, Boericke's, or Kent's. "To contravene Hahnemann's directions and teachings in every essential point, and to call themselves Hahnemannians par excellence, is quite unjustifiable, and is indeed absurd," Dudgeon argued. He did not mind practitioners making changes or departures in Hahnemann's rules, but that they did so and put themselves forward as "faithful interpreters" of Hahnemann was a travesty and a fraud. These so-called improvements should not be paraded as "Hahnemannian Homeopathy" but as "Hahnemannic principles."[32]

Despite Dudgeon's disparaging remarks, the editor of the *Homeopathic Recorder* cautioned readers not to be skeptical of the effects of the higher potencies. Admittedly, these potencies were as difficult to comprehend as the mind of Hamlet. The force inherent in the potencies, being little understood, had caused many to lose faith as the dynamization progressed into the higher centisimals. To help practitioners better understand their medical art, the editor explained that every elementary atom had a specific and distinctive energy. Thus, the atoms in a highly dynamized drug, such as mercury, contained a "certain potential energy" which became actualized only when the mass of the drug was separated. The separation of the drug force into its elemental atoms or molecules through dynamization turned low-potency mercury into a vital curative power. This was accomplished by attenuating a small amount in a medium of water, alcohol, or milk sugar and then succussing or triturating the mixture. When this occurred, the energy of the drug communicated its force to the medium which became in reality the drug itself "in a greatly diminished proportion, but a highly active state." The key was selecting a force that corresponded to the energy or vitality lost by the body in its disease state and freeing the needed amount of attenuated energy to respond to the lost vital energy of the body. What remained unclear was the number of succussions or triturations necessary to retain the molecular energy peculiar to the function it performed on the organism.[33]

The gulf between the materialistic mind of the allopath and the belief in the immaterial, spirit-like powers of medicinal substances held by the homeopath hurt the acceptance of homeopathy more than any other fact, explained Dr. J. H. Holloway of Illinois at a meeting of the IHA in 1910.[34] His remarks were testament to the "endless war" not only between allopathy and homeopathy, but also between and among members in the IHA and AIH. Hahnemann had very successfully practiced homeopathy with "material" doses before he discovered the principle of dynamization. For progressive members of the AIH, dynamization was a "science" that homeopathy could utilize, but was *not* homeopathy itself.[35]

"There can be no dispute among intelligent physicians about the evolution in the healing properties of a drug by the scientific method of attenuation," wrote John Prentice Rand, MD, in the *JAIH* in 1912, "but can we assent to the ultra proposition which affirms that the therapeutic properties of a drug can be communicated to an absolutely inert menstruum by the frictional contact induced by trituration or succussion and that this process may go on indefinitely?" To this question, he answered in the negative, preferring to believe that the cures ascribed to physical attenuations were the result of the *vis medicatrix naturae,* or something else. Rand explained that the theories advanced to explain the ultra attenuations "open[ed] the door to a maze of impossible considerations." Unless homeopaths could be sure that their attenuations contained some trace of medicinal substance they had no right to make any claims as to cures resulting from the medicine. He urged his colleagues to confine their practice to the use of actual attenuations and leave the vagaries of imaginary attenuations to others.[36]

Under pressure from critics to justify the effects of his high potencies, Dr. Bernhardt Fincke became a pioneer in the use of the galvanometer to detect the chemical action of medicines in the body. Using this device and a delicate astatic needle, he claimed that the human body acted as a conductor with an intensity that varied by sex, constitution, and condition of the organism. Other measurements of human energy included Walter J. Kilner's work on "The Human Aura" in *Science and Invention* (1921), which consisted of placing the individual before a darkened window to detect a "luminous mist" surrounding the body. Kilner likened this to the power of animals to follow an individual's "scent," and the belief in "Mephitis," or the ability to detect the "invisible emanations or rays given forth from the disintegration of actual particles" on the body. Other tests demonstrating the existence of highly attenuated potencies in the body involved the use of radium to photograph the 60th potency of bromide at the Boericke and Tafel Laboratories in Philadelphia.[37]

Homeopaths concluded from these various tests that in a condition of health, there was a harmonious interplay of energies in the body that vibrated at a specific rate. Disease, on the other hand, created a "disturbed resonance," or an "inharmonious play of the electronic forces." Every drug gave off the specific wave length and, when properly administered, correlated to the disease for which it was employed. The "homo-vibrations" which came from the drug were similar in kind to the disease and substantively different from the "hetero-vibrations" emanating from drugs of regulars that were dissimilar to the disease. It remained for the homeopathic school to thoroughly test its materia medica along these various lines by checking their response to electronic tests. Doing so would determine which drugs were or were not clinically effective. Potencies not found to show a response to the electronic tests were deemed clinically ineffective.[38]

X-RAYS

In the waning years of the nineteenth century, homeopathy's vitalist advocates found themselves drawn to the X-ray as a potential healing aid. In 1897, Dr. John B. Campbell X-rayed a flask of alcohol for a half-hour, believing that he was preparing an effective dynamization for patients suffering from dyscrasia (Hahnemannian miasm). Later that same year, the potentized X-ray was "proved" by the Brooklyn Hahnemannian Union under the supervision of Bernhardt Fincke and its results published in the *Proceedings of the International Hahnemannian Association.* Henry C. Allen wrote about the process in his *Materia Medica of the Nosodes and Provings of the X-Ray,* published in 1910. Despite optimistic claims, the remedy disappeared from the literature, partly because of the serious sclerotic and necrotic damage produced by the crude X-ray. Its toxic effect on the body was such that it suppressed the disease by overpowering the body's vitality. The Brooklyn provers, as it was soon discovered, developed side effects from the testing and several were so seriously injured they refused to take more than one dose. Nevertheless, Fincke advocated this remedy more than any other homeopath in his day and reported marvelous cures.[39]

Almost seventy years later, Federico Anaya-Reyes, MD, of Pueblo, Mexico, endorsed the use of this healing method as a health-restoring remedy in a variety of diseases. Instead of "awakening" the static energy with a tincture or solid substance by a dynamizing process, Anaya-Reyes used radiation to achieve the same end. Working with an appliance he called an "Electronic Attenuator X-O-Ray," he used radiation to provide gentle stimulation, thus "awakening organic resistance" in benign or malignant neoplasms.[40]

TISSUE REMEDIES

German physician Wilhelm Heinrich Schüssler's (1821-1897) method, popular among homeopaths at the turn of the twentieth century, consisted of reducing therapy to twelve cell-salts prepared in the form of powder and tablets triturated to the 3rd, 6th, or 12th potency and given dry on the tongue or dissolved in water. These vitalistic tissue remedies included calcarea fluoricum, calcarea phosphoricum, calcarea sulphuricum, ferrum phosphoricum, kali muriaticum, kali phosphoricum, kali sulphuricum, magnesia phosphoricum, naturm muriaticum, naturm phosphoricum, naturm sulphuricum, and silicea. Thought to be sufficient for all diseases, they were issued in a standard work on biochemistry in 1893.[41]

Homeopaths accepted the twelve salts with considerable zeal, but sometimes worried that physicians were content to confine themselves to these biochemic remedies alone and throw aside everything else in their materia medica. While critics credited Schüssler for his valued additions, they urged doctors not to fall into the error of "exclusivism, routinism or favoritism."[42] Nevertheless, William Boericke and Willis A. Dewey's well-known book, *The Twelve Tissue Remedies of Schüssler* (1893) became the basis for much of the popularity of the salts. The method was further complicated by the advertising of "Dr." George W. Carey whose "biochemic college" of which he was the founder, dean, and graduate—all in one year—traded on the remedies.[43]

Homeopaths adopted this biochemic therapy as a form of ultrascientific homeopathy, but Schüssler denied that the method was homeopathic. In the preface to his book, he wrote:

> Whenever small doses are mentioned the reader usually, at once, thinks of homeopathy; my therapy, however, is not homeopathic, for it is not founded on the law of similarity, but on the physiologic-chemical processes which take place in the human organism. By my method of cure the disturbances occurring in the motion of the molecules of the inorganic substances in the human body are directly equalized by means of homogenous substances, while homeopathy attains its curative ends in an indirect way by means of heterogeneous substances.[44]

Schüssler's therapy was based on facial diagnosis, that is, the ability to recognize the cardinal remedy in the face. Thus from the point of application, biochemistry and homeopathy were not comparable.[45] According to Leon Renard in 1940, homeopaths should reject this "infantile theory." Only the Law of Similia should be the guide of homeopaths.[46]

BACH FLOWERISM

Edward Bach (1886-1936) of England added to the canon of vitalistic remedies with his introduction of "flowerism," a system that used thirty-eight different flower essences to treat psychosomatic conditions.[47] According to Mechthild Scheffer, a lay practitioner and representative of the Bach Center in Germany, the flower and herbal remedies were used to correct the disharmony between the patient's soul and the mind, thus preparing the individual for recovery from any physical symptoms. The remedies helped build mental and spiritual growth and generally influenced the energy system within the patient. The method used was similar to that of classical homeopathy, anthroposophical medicine, and spagyric or herbal medicine, that is, the remedies worked by directly influencing the vitalistic element of the living organism. The flower essences, wrote Bach, "raise our vibrations and open up our channels for the reception of the Spiritual Self to flood our natures with the particular virtue we need, and wash out from us the fault that is causing the harm."[48] Each of the thirty-eight flowers embodied a certain "soul quality" or "energy wavelength" and when a particular flower remedy had the same energy frequency as the human soul quality, the two worked in rhythm to establish contact between the soul and personality that had become broken. Life then returned to an area where the disharmony existed. All plants were gathered in the wild and picked at the point of full maturity at which time they had a direct link to an individual's unconscious or higher self. The flower acted as an energy impulse and treated the patient, not the disease. The remedies were supplied in concentrated form in bottles and diluted in ethyl alcohol before use. The remedies were taken as drops on the tongue but also prescribed in compresses and in baths. Each remedy was associated with a set of emotional experiences or portrait. Bach believed that all diseases were of a mental origin and therefore the remedies must be prescribed on the basis of the mental indications of the patient.[49]

By the 1970s and 1980s, the use of flower essences as a healing art had grown exponentially as numerous individuals rediscovered Bach remedies and began expanding on his opus of essences. These included Lila Devi, the founder of the Master's Flower Essences; Steve Johnson's Alaskan Flower Essences; Molly Sheehan's Green Hope Essences; and Vasudeva and Kadambii Barnao's Living Essences, to mention a few. In all, some seven hundred flower essences have been tested and used on the basis of observation, conjecture, folklore, intuition, and trance channeling.[50]

SIXTH EDITION OF ORGANON

In 1921, the sixth edition of the *Organon* was published under the guidance of Richard Haehl (1873-1923) of Stuttgart and translated into English by Dr. William Boericke (1849-1929) of San Francisco.

Great interest accompanied the long-awaited edition. Both devotees and critics were curious as to what occupied the mind of Hahnemann in his last years. Had he changed his opinion on any of his fundamental principles? Had he further elucidated on his existing principles and philosophy? Had he formulated any new principles? Not surprisingly, most thought that he would focus on the issues of vitality, dynamism, and potentization, the last elements to be developed. They were not mistaken in their assumption in that Hahnemann enlarged upon the connection between mind and body. What enhanced the meanings behind much of what Hahnemann wrote were the subsequent inventions of the telegraph, telephone, electric dynamo, X-ray, phonograph, radio, the discovery of radium, and other advances which gave impulse and momentum to Hahnemann's dynamical principles.[51] Also among the important changes from the earlier 1833 edition was Hahnemann's recommendation for doses to be repeated daily, for months if deemed necessary. This advice proved troublesome for the high-potency wing of the profession who followed the practice of giving single doses at very long intervals.[52]

According to Stuart Close, up until the publication of this latest edition the vitalists within homeopathy had been fighting a "losing battle" with those who maintained that life could be explained from a purely chemical standpoint. However, chemistry could not explain all the vital processes. It broke down completely, he argued, when confronting the issue of "cerebration—the thinking process." In other words, no chemist could explain how "a chemical reaction or combination in the brain cells becomes a thought or a train of thought, a feeling, a sensation or an emotion." The same was true of the molecular, electrical, and ionic theories of vitality. In this latest edition of his *Organon,* Hahnemann finally took a definitive stand on vital force. It was clear that the ionic, atomic, molecular, cellular, mental, psychical, and even spiritual forces were simply "modes of action of the one primal, universal, all-inclusive power or principle . . . now identified as Life-and-Matter." This, Close reasoned, came from the theories of Herbert Spencer and linked homeopathy with all other true sciences. It also showed the direction in which further research should proceed. Until 1829, Hahnemann was a physicist and chemist in his thinking. In subsequent editions of *Organon,* he viewed the human organism as a "living, thinking, feeling unit and became a vitalist."[53]

ENERGY MEDICINES

In 1922, the *Homeopathic Recorder* published a paper by Doctors Benjamin C. Woodbury and Harry B. Baker on the dynamic power of infinitesimal dosages on the human organism. The molecular, atomic, and electronic structure of matter was now measurable, they explained, by way of electroscopes and spectroscopes, thus proving assertions made by Hahnemann as early as 1796 on the curative powers of small doses of medicine. The recognition of these infinitesimal dosages, they explained, marked the beginning of a process that eventually would confirm the effects of magnetism, electricity, crystallization, light, heat, affinity, and other forces on the body. These latter powers, referred to by Dr. Karl Baron Charles von Reichenbach (1788-1869) as the theory of "Od Force," "Odylic Force," or "Odic Force," were so subtle as to be perceived only by highly sensitized individuals. Nonetheless, according to the authors, these forces were now measurable and their results confirmed in experiments.[54]

The so-called OD theory (pronounced ode), or ergistic action of the homeopathic dose, had been introduced by Reichenbach as early as 1845. As explained by a Dr. Kirn of Berlin, only those who were truly sensitive could feel and see the OD. These so-called *sensitives* were defined as persons who were restless and given to insomnia; loved solitude; avoided crowds and handshaking; could not tolerate the fragrance of flowers; elected cold rather than warm food; avoided fats, sweets, and spices; refused tobacco, wine, and tea; preferred raw, unprepared foods; avoided constrictive clothing; were neurasthenic and susceptible to changes in the weather; and able to perceive peculiar forms of energy from light, magnets, electricity, crystals, and chemicals. An exaggerated sensitivity to stimuli is what made *sensitives* open to impressions not apprehended by the greater portion of mankind. This sensitivity was what accounted for the feud between the high and low potentists. According to Kirn, both accomplished genuinely homeopathic cures and the apparent confusion was due to the sensitive patient of "fine mentality" who only reacted to high potencies. Thus, the confusion among homeopaths and between homeopathy and regular medicine was actually brought about by the frequent mismatch of low- and high-potency drugs with sensitive and nonsensitive patients. The challenge for homeopaths was to learn how to identify these different types of patients and single them out for special treatment. Despite harsh criticism from the low-potency wing of homeopathy, the acceptance of the OD doctrine afforded homeopaths an important means of advancing treatment while, at the same time, reconciling their disparate belief systems.[55]

Yet another approach came when George Starr White of Los Angeles observed alterations of sound (vibratory rates) on certain pathological lesions, on drugs, and on other substances as the pitch changed polarity from east-west to north-south. Dr. Albert Abrams (1863-1924) of San Francisco took this information and, by introducing resistance coils between an individual and a substance, claimed to identify the existence of high dilutions of drugs in the blood and disease products.[56] All this had originally been put forth in his *New Concepts in Diagnosis and Treatment,* published in 1916. Abrams' avowed intention was to demonstrate the veracity of Hahnemannian theory regarding drug attenuation by demonstrating the existence of a traceable energy form in high-potency remedies. His findings satisfied homeopaths to the presence of drug substances in potencies as high as the 24th or 28th decimal. Similarly, in the Boericke and Tafel laboratories, tests gave positive photographic impressions with potencies of bromide as high as the 60th decimal, or the 20th centesimal. These laboratory demonstrations meant that physicians could be sure when prescribing a given potency of a drug that they were actually giving a preparation whose energy level or radioactivity had been recorded.[57]

An IHA committee headed by Guy Beckley Stearns, MD (1870-1947), professor of material medica at the New York Homeopathic Medical College and Flower Hospital, investigated the Abrams methods of diagnosis and treatment. Other members of the committee included Dr. Eugene Underhill, Dr. Henry Becker of Toronto, Dr. Harry B. Baker of Richmond, Dr. Benjamin C. Woodbury, Jr., of Boston, and Dr. Harvey Farrington of Chicago. Several of the committee members were in daily attendance at Abrams' clinics in San Francisco and there, along with other interested persons, sought to determine if there was any relation between the reactions of Abrams' oscilloclast and the curative remedy.[58] The committee had difficulty duplicating the experiments with the coils and, soon afterwards, the IHA dropped the use of Abrams's apparatus. The British Air Ministry was similarly interested in Abrams's claims but failed to find substantiating evidence.[59] As of 1924, no homeopathic organization had endorsed the Abrams theory of diagnosis and treatment. Although much talked about, his work remained at arm's length from the profession.[60]

The Foundation for Homeopathic Research, established in 1920 by Dr. Guy Beckley Stearns, developed connections with college clinics and associated hospitals to determine if high potencies had any effect on healthy animals.[61] The Foundation's objective was to approach the problems of homeopathy in a scientific manner. In its efforts to show the susceptibilities of drugs, the Foundation conducted experiments in the 1930s using guinea pigs and fruit flies. The guinea pig experiments were carried out over a period of two years, dosing 212 animals with ordinary salt in potencies ranging from the 30th to the 2000th. The general effect of the experiments was a marked slowing down in the rate of growth, a lessening of the frequency of birth, and the eventual extinction of virility. In the fruit-fly experiments, conducted by Dr. Mary Stark, arsenic was administered in the 30th and 200th potencies to various colonies of flies showing that these potencies freed certain colonies of their hereditary manifestations of tumor growths. Similar tests were carried out by Dr. W. J. S. Powers who worked with researchers in Eppendorf Hospital in Hamburg, Germany, on the effects of the tissue-salts in dilutions up to the 30th on paramecium concluded that the limit had not yet been reached.[62]

Also during the 1920s, Dr. William E. Boyd (1891-1955) a radiologist at Glasgow Homeopathic Hospital was engaged in the laboratory study on the nature and action of homeopathic potencies. Supported with a grant from the Beit Research Fund, he attempted to explain on a laboratory basis what it was in potentized medicines that produced results in homeopathic treatment. Using a spectroscope, fluorescent, and Geiger counter methods as well as his own device known as the emanometer, he experimented with low potencies of various homeopathic preparations to see if they were capable of identification. The experiments showed the activity of the 6X and 7X tinctures of radium bromide. This culminated in a report titled "Biochemical and Biological Evidence of the Activity of High Potencies," a document that stirred considerable response in the scientific world. The purpose of his research was to confirm that a substance prepared according to the homeopathic method was capable of affecting a biochemical process. To do this, he showed the effect of mercuric chloride, carried through 28X on the rate of breakdown of starch. Boyd's preparations were so dilute that most agreed no single molecule of the original drug could be present. Therefore, the power causing the effect had to be due to "some form of energy not yet understood." Although homeopaths had long posited the fact that substances prepared in this special way, either by serial dilution or mechanical shock, were active medicants, the scientific evidence had been lacking. Now, the evidence seemed to show that homeopaths were dealing with a form of energy that was as yet outside the scope of scientific medicine.[63]

In 1937, Boyd founded a Medical Research Institute to investigate the biological and physical properties of active substances when in dilute solution. After some fifteen years of research, he concluded that a drug diluted almost infinitely still retained a form of energy capable of affecting living cells. After his death, his son Dr. Hammish Boyd carried on his father's work. Throughout the 1960s, tests continued on Boyd's work, carried out by physical and biochemists, electricians, and other technical staff.[64]

During the late 1930s, articles explaining drug potentization drew on the quantum theory of German physicist Max Planck (1858-1947) who suggested that energy was released in bundles known as quanta and that these quanta varied with the frequency of the type of radiation of which they were a part. For homeopaths, this explained why a dose given to one individual might or might not evoke the same qualities or symptoms in another individual. This also explained why it took different potencies to affect different individuals, the healing response coming when the quantum of the drug and individual were most similar. Herbert A. Roberts' work *The Principles and Art of Cure by Homeopathy* (1942) made the point that the power or potency which perturbed the health of the prover would eventually turn out to be the same force that restored the health of the sick. Thus Hahnemann's Law of Similia was "interlocked" with the world of atoms, electrons, and protons within the fold of a universal concept—"the constitution of the far-flung cosmos of nature, and serve as the key to unlock the door to the great mystery of life."[65]

LAW OR PRINCIPLE

For more than a century, homeopaths had fought a persistent battle over the use of the letters "a" and "e" in the spelling of *similia similibus curantur* and *similia similibus curentur.* The advocates of *curantur* were generally found among Hahnemannians like Constantine Hering and Adolphe Lippe who, adhering strictly to the teachings of the *Organon,* viewed the Law of Similia as part of the fundamental or natural law of nature. For them, the verb was correctly written in the indicative mood to demonstrate how firm, sure, and confident Hahnemann and his followers adhered to their standard. The champions of *curentur,* on the other hand, were found chiefly among more liberal homeopaths such as Richard Hughes (1836-1902) who advocated the use of low-potency remedies, and Robert E. Dudgeon who interpreted the law as more permissive, that is, let likes be treated by likes.[66]

Toward the end of the nineteenth century, when homeopaths were planning to erect a monument of Hahnemann at Scott's Circle in the nation's capital, they concluded that *curantur* implied too much and therefore decided to provide a more limiting connotation. In its place, they substituted *curentur,* suggesting "they may be cured."[67] The proposal to make the change came from Dr. James H. McClelland (1845-1913) who claimed to have taken the spelling from the fourth edition of the *Organon.*[68] Others who supported the change noted that *curentur* could be found in the 1836 American edition of the *Organon* and in the unauthorized German sixth edition edited by Dr. Ernest Arthur Lutz (1813-1870) in 1865. According to Wilhelm Ameke in his *History of Homeopathy* (1885), Hahnemann himself used the spelling *curentur.* As a result, William Tod Helmuth, Sr. (1833-1902), chief surgeon at the New York Homeopathic Medical College and Hospital and dean from 1893 to 1902, announced *curentur* as the official spelling at the AIH session held in Atlantic City, New Jersey, in June 1899. On June 23, 1900 the monument was officially dedicated.[69]

The difference between "similars are cured" and "similars may be cured" was significant for believers and critics alike in the early decades of the twentieth century. In articles written for the AIH, authors typically used the spelling of *curantur,* while the editorial staff preferred the *curentur* spelling.[70] In 1909, when the AIH called for a change in the spelling of the word in its constitution and bylaws, the Hahnemannians objected.[71] As explained by G. H. Thacher, associate editor of the *Homeopathic Recorder,* students in homeopathic colleges had been taught that *curantur* was a method of cure which science had made obsolete. As instructed by their "left wing" faculty, they had come to believe that many of the provings were "trash" if not the "ravings of unscientific minds." For Thacher it was the proving of the remedy which marked the distinction between allopathy and homeopathy. The proving of the remedies, singly, and on healthy individuals, represented the primary difference. Issues of similarity, size of dose, potency, and repetition were secondary. This dispute between liberals and conservatives marked yet another skirmish in their protracted warfare.[72]

In 1935, Harvey Farrington, MD (1872-1957), a pupil of Kent and author of *Homeopathy and Homeopathic Prescribing* (1955), presented a paper on the subject to the IHA's Bureau of Homeopathic Philosophy. In it, he attempted to bring an end to the controversy by suggesting that the use of the two spellings was a matter of "individual opinion or choice." However, if desiring to know Hahnemann's preference, it was *similia similibus curentur.* Hahnemann never had written *curantur* in any of his exhaustive works.[73]

In 1988, the *JAIH* challenged homeopaths worldwide to examine *similia similibus curentur* to determine whether it should be a law, a principle, or merely a useful guide in the treatment of the sick. Was Hahnemann's language more like a law, meaning "likes will be cured by likes," as opposed to "let likes be cured by likes?" Skeptics pointed out that Hahnemann, who had been an excellent linguist who framed his language carefully, never referred to the former.[74]

Randall Neustaedter, OMD (b. 1949), who started the Bay Area Homeopathic Study Group in 1972, held that the law of similars was the "only curative mechanism of therapeutics." Nevertheless, he knew from both Hahnemann and from Kent that the law had limitations. For example, surgical cases were outside the realm of medical therapy and certain cases were incurable. Other conditions, he was willing to admit, required allopathic intervention. Whether the law of similars always applied and whether it was the only curative method was for Neustaedter something as yet inconclusive and made even more difficult by the principle of individualization which carried any number of idiosyncrasies into a particular case. As to whether the law of similars was the only method of cure, he feared that homeopaths who viewed the law of similars as "sovereign" were reluctant to consider using another appropriate therapy. This, he reasoned, presented a problem. He concluded that it was impossible for homeopaths to answer the question respecting the Law of Similia unless they were willing to look at other curative or palliative therapies.[75]

Notwithstanding Neustaedter's concerns, Harris Coulter, PhD, author of *Divided Legacy* (1973-77) had few if any doubts of the Law of Similia's universal application. "I am sad to see homeopaths once again engaged in 'threshing straw'," he complained. Coulter found that the continuing discussion was but a reflection of "the physician's reluctance to be bound by a rule which constricts his freedom of choice." Nevertheless, a law was a law. "Unless the law of similars is maintained as an ideal toward which we must always strive, we will fall into the same routines as the allopathic majority, and the patients, as usual, will pay the penalty."[76]

William Shevin, MD, responded to the question by suggesting that the similia was "probably" a law but that homeopathy was not in a position at the time to answer it definitively. There were too many steps at which error could occur to be so sure.

> The law of similars is the sole scientific basis of homeopathic practice. I do not mean to suggest by this that it is sacrosanct—it should be continually subjected to scrutiny and verification. I do not think that the information presented to date can support serious doubts as to the standing of the law of similars. It works much more often than it appears to fail . . . the failure is much more likely to be in ourselves (or in the incurability of the patient) than in the underlying principles.[77]

In responding to the challenge, Ahmed Currim, MD, suggested that just as in physics where Newton's laws were refined and then superceded by more general laws, so it was entirely possible that the Law of Similia would be superceded by a more general law which encompassed similia. Until that time came, however, it was appropriate to view *similia similibus curentur* as "a natural law of healing" and which "will lead to a clearer knowledge of the science of therapeutics as it is applied to more disease phenomena." Part of the problem in confronting the similia had to do with the "uncontrollable variables" which often inhibited the law's proper application. For example, a practitioner may have insufficient medical training or insufficient knowledge of homeopathy and of the *Organon*. Then again, the practitioner may have failed to perform a complete case-taking, physical exam, or laboratory tests; he may similarly have incomplete knowledge of the symptom-complex; have chosen an incorrect potency; or drawn a wrong conclusion from the literature.[78]

Whether the law of similars was a "natural law" of unvarying truth at all times and in all circumstances, or a principle or rule that was "deductively valid but not always applicable," or simply a "practical guideline, often useful but not in any sense binding," were questions that ruminated through the literature as late as the 1980s. Homeopath Richard Moskowitz, MD, who received his medical education at New York University School of Medicine and who taught regularly at the National Center for Homeopathy, parted company with many of his colleagues on the law of similars, noting that "even the laws of mathematics and physics are valid only within the formal conditions specified by them." He knew from experience that other nonhomeopathic treatments often served a useful purpose and therefore found it impossible to accept Hahnemann's implication that homeopathy was the only form of healing and that all other methods were in error. This made any "meaningful synthesis of the health care system impossible," he wrote. Nevertheless, he saw the Law of Similia "as close to a natural law as we are likely to get."[79]

* * *

There seemed to be no end to the expansiveness of esoteric homeopathy's beliefs and practices. Forged between physical healing and the higher spiritual planes, its dimensions appeared limitless as it searched for causal agencies connecting the human mind with the cosmic order. Disillusioned with the static conceptual categories of Enlightenment rationality, Hahnemannians exercised their metaphysical imaginations to articulate a philosophy of vitalism that would bring physical events under some providential law or purpose. However, as critic Rudolph Rabe of the *Homeopathic Recorder* observed, esoteric or high-potency Hahnemannianism had transformed homeopathy into a "blind fanaticism" that was preventing it from advancing as a legitimate branch of medicine. "We of the homeopathic school, or what is left of it, must keep our feet upon firm ground and must build our theories upon a foundation of solid fact," Rabe advised. "We must interpret homeopathy in the light of scientific advancement; for homeopathy, being true, can have no quarrel with modern science."[80]

Chapter 3

The Laity Speaks Out

The spread of homeopathy in the United States came from two sources: one professional, the other, lay. The professional route went from physician to student by means of preceptorships and didactic education, and from one physician to another through formal and informal contacts. Through the first half of the nineteenth century, the greatest number of these professionals came as converts from regular medicine. By the second half of the century, the medically trained homeopath came principally from one of sixty-nine colleges organized between 1835 and 1935. The other route, via the laity, was equally important. Lay advocates were often owners of books on domestic treatment and accompanying boxes of attenuated medicines. Anxious to support their new-found healing system, and convinced of its efficacy over mainstream medicine, they used their money, power, and influence to obtain equity before the law; raise money to build hospitals and clinics; and establish departments of homeopathy in universities. In almost all their endeavors, however, they deferred medical judgment to the academically trained physician.

In the aftermath of Flexner's classic *Medical Education in the United States and Canada* (1910), the increased powers given to the AAMC and the AMA's Council on Medical Education, the fiscal and legal implications of medical rankings, the abolition of separate examining boards, and the slow but steady decline in the numbers of homeopathic colleges, the laity became more vocal in expressing their concerns over the future of their healing system. Not surprisingly, many took exception to what they perceived to be the spread of adjectival medicine within their remaining colleges and the slow but incremental homogenization of homeopathy into mainstream medicine. Convinced that the faculties of these schools had been beguiled by the promises of reductionist medicine and the catholicity of practice, they began taking steps to return homeopathy to Hahnemann's original principles.

AMERICAN FOUNDATION FOR HOMEOPATHY

Established in June 1921 by a group of high potency physicians affiliated with the International Homeopathic Association (IHA) and led by Dr. Julia M. Green (1871-1963), the American Foundation for Homeopathy (AFH) represented the first real effort to counteract the demise of the colleges with the establishment of postgraduate education. The AFH was organized around three overriding principles: (1) the future of homeopathy depended on the cooperation of physicians and laity; (2) instruction in homeopathy should be postgraduate in nature; and (3) nationwide publicity among the laity was essential to ensure homeopathy's "rightful place in the world." The foundation justified its work having concluded that the existing medical organizations were no longer serving the profession or the people in the manner originally intended; that the remaining homeopathic colleges were closing due to reasons both internal and external; that few state licensing boards continued to have homeopathic representation; and that applicants for licenses to practice medicine were no longer tested on their prescribing abilities.[1] The Foundation's offices were located at 1724 H Street in the District of Columbia. Initial trustees included Doctors Alonzo E. Austin (1868-1948) of New York; Cyrus M. Boger (1861-1935) of West Virginia; George E. Dienst (1858-1932) of Chicago; Frederica E. Gladwin (1856-1931) of Philadelphia; Julia M. Green (1871-1963) of Washington, DC; Julia C. Loos (1869-1929) of Pittsburgh; and Frank W. Patch (1862-1923) of Boston. Its single lay trustee was George E. Fleming of Washington, DC.

Although a cursory view of the literature convinced many that homeopathy was either dead or dying, Julia M. Green, a graduate of Wellesley (1893) and Boston University Medical School (1898), and one of the leading spirits of homeopathy, challenged the assumption, sure in her mind that the fundamentals of homeopathy were growing in popularity every day. The power of the infinitesimal had become a familiar term thanks to the influence of the media. Reflecting the pulse of the Progressive Era in politics and culture, Green predicted a continuing trend toward reform in America. The value and power of the single individual was more important than ever before. Green predicted that, in time, homeopathy would gain vision, unanimity of purpose, and efficiency.[2] Green dedicated herself to resolving what she perceived was a serious misunderstanding between homeopathic physicians and the laity. This misunderstanding included personal jealousies, a proliferation of dubious remedies, and medical politics. Green called for both sides to come together. Instead of fighting among themselves, she urged homeopaths to correlate the Law of Similia with the latest developments in physics, chemistry, religion, social welfare, philanthropy, hygiene, criminology, eugenics, physical training, mental training, and diet.[3] A Kentian in medicine and a Unitarian in religion, she followed in the footsteps of her mentor, Dr. Frederica Gladwin (1856-1931) of Philadelphia, and taught Kent's *Repertory* at the Post Graduate Summer School sponsored by the AFH.[4]

In developing its educational program, the AFH quickly discovered a division within its ranks on whether the organization should be training physicians only or expanding its reach to include interested laypersons. Having agreed to include laypersons, the question then became whether or not they should be taught the use of remedies. The AFH organized its postgraduate teaching first in the District of Columbia, and later in Boston, where classes were provided at the School of Fine Arts on Beacon Street. Students came from Sweden, Switzerland, Yugoslavia, East Africa, India, and the United States. Its six-week course required the reading of Hahnemann's *Organon* (1833), Kent's *Lectures in Homeopathic Philosophy* (1900), portions of Stuart Close's *Genius of Homeopathy* (1924), Alexis Carrel's *Man, the Unknown* (1938), and Dr. Herbert A. Roberts' *The Principles and Art of Cure by Homeopathy* (1942). The lectures covered such topics as vital force as expressed in health, disease, recovery, and cure; the relation of sickness to the patient; susceptibility; suppression; palliation; disease classification; and manifestations of latent disease. There was also a course of study in the materia medica; case-taking and its relation to repertory study, particularly of Kent and Boenninghausen; and practical instruction in case management, including acute and chronic patients. The course even included clinical medicine carried out at the clinics of Dr. R. W. Spalding at the Massachusetts Memorial Hospital and the Union Rescue League.[5] Among the many students enrolled in the training were Dr. M. Gururaju and Dr. P. Narayanaraju of India, reflecting the multicultural nature of the program and the extent of its international influence.[6] The AFH organized the program on the dormitory plan where students were kept isolated from outside distractions. Doing so allowed the teachers to provide a course equal to what students might obtain in a single year of undergraduate education.[7]

In Los Angeles, Doctors A. Dwight Smith (1885-1980), W. E. Jackson, and Carl H. Enstam offered a postgraduate course to all medical doctors, including osteopaths. The course met one night per month but remained unsponsored and offered no credential or certificate. In San Francisco, postgraduate education was offered through Hahnemann Hospital while, further to the north, a laity organization known as the Northwest Foundation for Homeopathy devoted its time and resources to postgraduate education in anticipation of when the legislature might create a medical school at the University of Washington.[8]

Postgraduate instruction was available in Washington, D.C., from 1922 to 1927 where Dr. Green conducted courses open to any MD or undergraduate after the junior year. Postgraduate instruction was also offered to physicians at Metropolitan Hospital on Welfare Island in New York in 1927; at Forest Hills, Massachusetts, where Dr. Alonzo J. Shadman (1877-1960), a graduate of Boston University Medical School, headed a group; in Boston, Massachusetts, from 1928 to 1937 where Dr. Herbert A. Roberts (1868-1950), a pupil of Close, conducted summer courses before the Second World War, and where classes were reactivated again in 1946; in Spring Valley, New York, from 1939 to 1941; and in Chicago, Illinois, where Dr. Harvey Farrington (1872-1957), a pupil of Kent and president of the IHA in 1922, offered correspondence courses for those unable to attend in person.[9] In addition, the board of trustees of the former Cleveland Pulte Medical College used the school's remaining endowment to sponsor postgraduate courses in homeopathy and correspondence courses as well. Although lacking the official sanction and supervision of the AIH, the trustees nonetheless continued with their educational efforts.[10] Postgraduate schools of homeopathy, including several open to the laity, also operated in Belgium, France, Germany, Holland, India, Italy, Spain, Mexico, Switzerland, and Great Britain.[11]

As directed by Dr. Kenneth A. McLaren, the Bureau of Instruction of the AFH held back from giving laity instruction in diagnosis, laboratory methods or analysis, and discussions as to the relative virtues of different methods of treatment. Rather, the aim of the bureau was to furnish a true concept of the homeopathic law of cure, the nature of chronic disease, and the homeopathic method of cure. Despite these self-imposed limitations, the AIH refused to work with the AFH because their physician members feared the increased role of the laity in the AFH, the often extravagant claims of its high potency members, and the AFH's decision to admit osteopaths, dentists, and veterinarians as members.[12]

Postgraduate work was on the minds of homeopaths in the late 1930s, particularly in the wake of the Great Depression and the failure of the AIH to establish any new colleges or raise sufficient endowment to support its two remaining colleges—Hahnemann of Philadelphia and New York Homeopathic. The AIH had not set forth an official statement, but the need for postgraduate education was the topic of its Five-Year Plan Committee and its Education Committee, both of which viewed it as necessary for the future of homeopathy, its philosophy, and the scientific application of its principles.[13] In 1941, following the decision of the AMA to no longer include sectarian schools on its approved list of medical schools, the AIH officially endorsed the concept by joining forces with the Bureau of Instruction in the AFH and pledging itself to support the bureau's program. In making this endorsement, American homeopaths officially joined other countries in endorsing postgraduate instruction, having concluded that mixing homeopathy with undergraduate studies did not work.[14]

When enrollments declined in the mid-1950s, the AFH replaced its six-week course with a two-week program in the hope that the shorter period would attract larger classes. Students were housed at the Millersville State Teachers' College eight miles southwest of Lancaster, Pennsylvania. Accommodation in its dormitories cost $6 per day and the fee for the course itself was $100. The course covered the principles of homeopathy, materia medica, clinical homeopathy, and repertorization (principally the books of Kent and Boenninghausen). Instructors included Dr. Ray W. Spalding of Boston; Dr. Elizabeth Wright Hubbard (1896-1967) of New York City; Dr. Eugene Underhill, Jr. (b. 1913) of Philadelphia; Dr. Allan D. Sutherland (1897-1980) of

Battleboro; and Dr. Garth W. Boericke (1893-1968) of Philadelphia.[15] During the 1960s, postgraduate homeopathy was also taught in New York, Connecticut, Ohio, and at the Southern Homeopathic Convention in Atlanta, at the Pan American in Bermuda, and at the annual conventions of the AIH.

Despite good intentions, the AFH's efforts to salvage homeopathy through postgraduate education proved disappointing, introducing few new physicians into the field. Even the admission of osteopaths, dentists, and veterinarians failed to make a significant difference in numbers. With renewed interest in alternative medicine in the 1960s, the AFH opened its classes to chiropractors, naturopaths, registered nurses, medical assistants, and paraprofessionals.

In 1972, the Millersville State College program opened its doors to the laity for a one-week course of instruction in homeopathy and homeotherapeutics. The teaching staff included Dr. Henry Williams, Director of the National Center for Homeopath's division of education; Dr. Ruth Rogers of Daytona Beach, Florida; Dr. David Wember of McLean, Virginia; Dr. Harris Coulter who spoke on the history and philosophy of homeopathy; and pharmacist John Bornemann. When physicians objected to attending classes with the laity, the courses were segregated, giving physicians the opportunity to delve more deeply into areas of practice.[16]

As much as Julia Green placed the future of true homeopathy in the hands of the laity, other academically educated homeopaths doubted that the laity would be able to live by the principles of the Law of Similia, the single remedy, and the minimum dose. They feared that while the laity talked as though they were homeopaths, they actually mixed, combined, and compounded medicines in an unscientific and wholly unhomeopathic manner in order to address particular symptoms.[17] Within the AIH, this bifurcated view was played out between the members of its Council on Medical Education and the Council on Legislation as they struggled for a definition of medicine. The former intended the definition to cover all practitioners, both liberal and conservative, while the latter excluded all who were not practitioners in the classical sense.[18]

Despite the continued opposition of the few remaining homeopathic physicians to the intrusion of the laity into the theory and practice of their medicine, homeopathy's high potency advocates turned more and more to the laity for support and direction. As will be seen, the decision had a distasteful edge as this broadened democracy came with a spirit of self-sufficiency, an ill-tempered indifference to the licensed physician, and an unapologetic willingness to resurrect old heresies. Millenarian in spirit, the laity broke with homeopathy's Baconian roots by expressing an uninhibited affection for the oracular and mystical side of healing.

LAYMEN'S LEAGUES

Under Julia Green's leadership, the AFH began forming a grassroots network of so-called laymen's leagues in the 1920s to keep homeopathy alive for future generations. Their intent was fourfold: to learn what homeopathy was; to spread knowledge of it among the people; to find physicians willing to study homeopathy in a postgraduate structure; and to raise money for work on behalf of the leagues. To accomplish these tasks, Green sent letters to homeopaths across the country, informing them of the purposes of the AFH and of its desire to combine the interests of physicians and the laity in the spread of homeopathic beliefs. Her goal was to form leagues in every city or town where homeopathy was still robust.[19]

Green's Bureau of Publicity published a file on current homeopathic literature and sent out bulletins titled "Laymen's Leagues" which were distinct from those intended for physicians. Items of interest included the state of knowledge concerning homeopathy; history of homeopathy's growth to the present time; stories for young people; reasons for the laity to work on behalf of homeopathy; relevant statistics; a directory of physicians for travelers; case reports; definitions; list of leagues with membership and activities; and announcements of postgraduate classes. The bureau also published a set of questions and answers for the laity, as well as a set of cures written for their use.[20]

The idea for the leagues was not entirely new. As early as the 1890s, Dr. Stuart Close of Brooklyn had begun assembling interested patients for talks and discussions concerning the principles of homeopathy. This group eventually formed into the Homeopathic Laymen's League of New York and proceeded to arrange for regular talks designed to educate the laity in the principles of homeopathy and to join them in regional and national projects in support of the profession. Eventually other homeopathic physicians, including Mary Florence Taft and Rufus L. Thurston in Boston; George E. Dienst in Aurora, Illinois; Julia C. Loos in Pittsburgh; and Frederica E. Gladwin in Philadelphia found ready-made audiences among their more active patients.

The first league to be established under the auspices of the AFH was the Homeopathic Laymen's League of Washington, D.C., which organized as a group of fifty men and women on December 6, 1924 under the leadership of Dr. Green. Its bylaws placed the league under the guidance of the foundation's Bureau of Publicity and its stated objectives were to study homeopathic principles; encourage the study by medical students of the practice of homeopathy; provide financial aid through the Ada Putnam Lawton Scholarship to students attending the Post-Graduate School of the AFH; administer and support the scholarship fund; and contribute financially to the bureau. The league held monthly meetings in private homes with speakers that included both physicians and laypersons. It sponsored an annual banquet with guest speakers from Canada, England, Switzerland, and India. In addition, the league conducted study classes for the laity and sponsored the publication of booklets for distribution. Dues were $2 per year.[21]

A Laymen's League also formed in New York City under the presidency of Mrs. Elizabeth Close, meeting monthly at the Woodstock Hotel, with about fifty members at each meeting. When members expressed concern over the lack of doctors to teach and practice the principles and cures of homeopathy, the league set out to increase the number of "intelligent laymen" who were willing to learn what simple homeopathic remedies could accomplish—remedies found in their own home and prescribed for themselves when no physician was available. In other words, the league set out to provide an intelligent group of patients ready to cooperate with physicians but still manage on their own when necessary.[22]

Other leagues formed in Philadelphia, Boston, Seattle, and Southern California. In an address before the Homeopathic Laymen's League of Philadelphia in 1944, layperson Max Shernoff recalled his earliest connection with homeopathy, his curiosity at reading the *Organon,* his conversion to the Law of Similia, and his use of a domestic medical book and box of medicines.[23] In Glendale, California, the Homeopathic Laymen's Association of Southern California worked with the local homeopathic medical society to establish chairs of homeopathy in regular medical schools and to establish a postgraduate school.[24]

Increasingly, American homeopaths viewed their lay organizations as key to the future. During the 1920s, the AFH's Bureau of Publicity carried out an educational campaign on matters of prevention, personal health, and public welfare. In 1926, even the AIH considered the publication of a lay magazine as a means of communicating to a broader reading audience. As evidence of this turn of events, the AIH encouraged the publication of the *Central Journal of Homeopathy* (1920-26), a health magazine written in nonmedical language and distributed through the Women's Homeopathic League of the Ohio State Homeopathic Society.[25] "Whatever is to become of homeopathy depends upon what the laymen thinks of it," observed J. Clifford Hayner, editor of the *JAIH* in 1935. In a period where allopaths outnumbered homeopaths ten to one, it was the laity who represented the "deciding factor" in the future. "Abstract theories and broad claims based upon homeopathic achievements in the past will mean little," Hayner added. "Only the living status of homeopathy and the total number of votes then at hand will count." For this reason, it was essential for homeopathy to advertise itself in the daily press and radio; impress the "incomparable exactitude" with which homeopathic prescriptions met the special needs of patients; and reawaken public esteem in homeopathy's teachings and accomplishments. For all of these tasks, the laity offered a valuable and unique service.[26]

With the active support of the laity, and on the advice of a consulting firm contracted to assess the potential role of laypersons, the AIH formed the National Homeopathic Lay Council in 1931 to develop and extend the knowledge and practice of homeopathy as a therapeutic art. To accomplish this objective, the council was empowered to assist medical schools, hospitals, dispensaries, students and teachers in the collection of data; support publications and conferences; raise endowment funds; and establish branch offices in the various states.[27]

In September 1936, Julia Green introduced a two-page section titled "For the Layman" into issues of the *Homeopathic Recorder.* The topics addressed in her column covered a host of issues: the value of homeopathy in surgery; scientific confirmation of homeopathic theory; the life of Hahnemann; explanations of triturations and potencies; modern conceptions of homeopathy; comparisons of homeopathy with allopathy; homeopathic treatment for the common cold; homeopathy and germ theory; the laity's view of physicians; the laity's obligation to homeopathy; vaccination; mind and emotions as factors in disease; homeopathic philosophy; and the conception of the unity of man and the world. Explaining that times had changed and that it was important to acquaint the laity with the "why and wherefore" of medicine, she identified two specific purposes for her department. *First,* laypersons should understand the principles of homeopathy, how best to select a competent physician, and answer for themselves and for friends the questions most often asked about homeopathy and its form of treatment. *Second,* laypersons became better patients by understanding what to report to their physicians and how to cooperate in treatment. To support her work on the section, Green asked the laity to submit questions, make suggestions and comments, and to criticize freely.[28]

Unlike others who were genuinely fearful of the direction being taken to include the laity in matters heretofore reserved for licensed physicians, Green chose not to dilute her communications with the laity. Instead, she treated them with the same courtesy she addressed to physicians. Arguing, for example, that some patients were overly sensitive to odors, others to certain noises, and still others to light or music, she explained that these susceptibilities were important in choosing the correct remedy. To be successful, a homeopathic remedy had to be "tuned to the plane of the patient's susceptibility to it." Essentially, a remedy must meet the situation "on the same plane as the disorder."[29] Sickness began in the "innermost" of the patient and flowed outward. Disease did not lie in the patient's environment, or in bacteria, or in anything from without. The intrinsic cause lay in the patient himself. In making this point, Green explained that it was important not to confuse sickness with its expression since the expression of a disease may show only on the skin.[30] Green also used her column to introduce the idea of "vibration" as understood from discoveries in physics, chemistry, biology, astronomy, and even music to help explain homeopathic phenomena. Vibrations were everywhere—"disorderly, producing disease, discord, ugliness, misunderstanding—orderly, producing health, harmony, beauty, understanding, wisdom."[31] Just as harmony in music is produced by thirds, sixths, octaves, etc., so potencies acted best with a "rhythmic scale" of intervals between them.[32]

CONCERNS

To be sure, not all of homeopathy's leadership was favorably disposed to the methods taken by Julia Green and her associates to educate the laity. One prominent naysayer was Stuart Close of the *Homeopathic Recorder* who cautioned readers that there was a right way and a wrong way to educate the public and raise the morale of the homeopathic profession. Unfortunately, he believed that the methods used to advance homeopathy on a large scale had been carried out "by means and methods which have been anything but modest and far from dignified." Clearly, he was not pleased with the "propagandistic campaign" of Green since she had "unwisely implied and mistakenly assumed" that the public regarded homeopaths as incompetent. The psychological effect of this suggestion, he reasoned, had resulted in an unfavorable image of homeopathy. "Instead of taking it for granted and assuming that the public regards all physicians recognized and licensed by the State as competent in general to practice medicine," Green's approach suggested the contrary and "tended to arouse doubt and uncertainty about the competency of the men who thus drew public attention to themselves." Better to instruct the public in the theory, principles, and scope of homeopathy than to place it in a reactive mode of defending itself against false charges. A well-written platform of principles and practical demonstrations in hospitals, clinics, and dispensaries would have been preferable to its current program of activity. Given the public's skepticism toward such other nonmedical practices as Christian Science, osteopathy, and chiropractic, it was important to demonstrate the thorough grounding of homeopathy in the traditional foundations of medicine. Better to follow the lead of the AMA and big business in placing its publicity needs in the hands of experts. "There has been altogether too much amateur work in this department," he stated.[33]

Admitting that Laymen's Leagues were important organizations and essential for the future of homeopathy, the editor of the *Homeopathic Recorder* insisted that they required the guidance of physicians and the "supervision and endorsement" of homeopathic medical associations. The leagues' function was to create interest among the public and encourage a demand for physicians in the art of healing. However, it was not the function of these leagues to teach materia medica or to give the laity instruction in the application of remedies in the treatment of the sick. Certainly talks on health, preventive medicine, and diet were all within the bounds of these leagues. Beyond that, they should operate in close consultation with the homeopathic physician. "The Leagues can advertise homeopathy in a quiet, inoffensive and effective way but it must not be haphazard, isolated attempts; it must be organized, planned action."[34]

In an effort to skirt criticism from laypersons that the IHA lacked confidence in their abilities and, at the same time, ensure that the leagues kept within proper boundaries, the editor suggested that the IHA appoint a Laymen's League Committee with supervisory powers over the leagues. Each league should select one of its members to a Central Board of Governors. Most feared by the IHA was the possibility that the leagues would extend their power without guidance from trained physicians. Properly supervised and encouraged, there was almost no limit to their possibilities; but improperly supervised, they posed an impediment to the integrity of homeopathy's theory and practices.[35] In his president's address before the IHA in 1937, Eugene Underhill, Jr., admitted that the ideal role for the leagues had not yet evolved. He even suggested that another name might be more appealing to members (i.e., Hahnemannian Round Table Groups) in districts where there were medical colleges and students interested enough to attend meetings and learn case-taking, materia medica, and repertory analysis. He said, "It is still possible to win converts if we go about it in the right spirit and in a friendly and inoffensive way."[36]

Few were as sympathetic with the growing preponderance of the laity in homeopathy's future as Carl H. Enstam of California. Having decided that postgraduate education had failed in its mission to educate licensed physicians and that, as a result, hundreds of pseudo-homeopaths were practicing a crude eclectic form of homeopathy, he decided to place his hope in the power and persuasiveness of the laity.[37] Believing that homeopathy must plan its reconstruction more carefully, Enstam urged aggressive publicity along with the organization and education of the laity. "We must encourage a nationwide organization of laymen," argued Enstam, thereby bringing patrons and practitioners together on a common ground. "Homeopathy must go to the laity," he concluded. "The moment lay interest is aroused and awakened to the possibilities of homeopathy, an irresistible force will have been set to work which will no longer tolerate arbitrary medication."[38]

Layperson training in emergency medicine assumed strategic importance in towns and cities during the Second World War when most physicians were called away to serve in the Armed Forces. Often in the night when acute sickness struck, the "domestic physician" reached out to a book on homeopathic remedies and used a few doses of aconite, belladonna, or some other plant remedy until a professional doctor could be called.[39]

While the leagues continued to remain active through the 1940s, state and county homeopathic societies were neglected. The last remaining medical colleges with chairs of homeopathy also experienced difficulties. In the absence of physicians with homeopathic experience, they underwent extensive changes in organization and training, with little homeopathy being added to their programs.[40]

By the mid-1950s, lay societies included the Women's National Homeopathic League; the Homeopathic Laymen's League of Washington, D.C.; the Chicago Homeopathic Laymen's League; the Boston Homeopathic Society; the Homeopathic Laymen's League of New York; the Women's Homeopathic League of Pennsylvania; the Central Pennsylvania Homeopathic Medical Auxiliary; the Northwest Homeopathic Foundation; and the Texas Homeopathic League. In addition to these organizations, there were thirty-seven state and sectional societies, and ten national and international associations. By 1968, there were eleven chapters of the Federation of Laymen's Leagues operating in the United States; by 1975, there were sixteen fully functioning organizations.[41]

Increasingly, lay societies and their leaders demanded larger and larger roles in the profession. In an open letter to the profession in 1956, Mrs. Elinore C. Peebles and Mrs. Edith S. Capon of Boston expressed concern with the ever-diminishing numbers of doctors and hospitals and urged the greater involvement of their lay associations. With a stronger partnership between professional homeopaths and lay groups, a more effective and coordinated strategy was possible. "Laymen . . . can do little to initiate worthwhile projects as goals toward which to strive without the leadership of the profession," they explained. They noted that lay societies had pleaded for a greater role in the affairs of the association as early as 1914 and that their active participation in the preservation of homeopathy had prevented its disappearance.[42]

At the same time the leagues were demanding a larger role in homeopathy's organizations, they were also beginning to break ranks. In the early 1950s, for example, President Elizabeth Close of the Homeopathic Laymen's League of New York reported having received requests from members for the inclusion of spiritual and religious leaders as well as astrologers as potential lecturers. While she did not feel these groups deserved notice or a place on the lecture calendar, especially when it was easy to attach the word "cult" to their activities, the very indication of these influences created further tension between the professional homeopath and the laity, a tension that would intensify in the decades to come.[43]

The first meeting of delegates to the Layman's Bureau of the AIH took place in June 1957 with twenty-six in attendance. Chairing the meeting was Dr. Arthur H. Grimmer who led the group through an agenda that included the clear and unmistakable role and responsibility of the AIH; the supporting role of the Layman's Bureau in helping to unify but not dominate; publications that the AIH would edit *before* publishing; and recognition that laypersons wishing to form leagues should do so only under the guidance of AIH doctors.[44]

It is interesting to note that homeopaths were not alone in their decision to seek a closer partnership with the laity. While both New York and Boston radio stations were broadcasting programs to answer the need of laypersons for information, news, and comment on homeopathy, the AMA began publication in 1950 of its own lay magazine, *Today's Health,* intended to serve the American family. The publication continued until 1976 when it was succeeded by *Family Health.*[45]

THE LAYMAN SPEAKS

In 1926, the AFH introduced *Homeopathic Survey,* a quarterly magazine devoted to the cause of pure homeopathy by means of postgraduate courses in homeopathic philosophy and materia medica, therapeutics, and repertory analysis. The magazine was the inspiration of Dr. Benjamin C. Woodbury of Boston, who later became president of the IHA. The magazine was divided into four bureaus: investigation, research and demonstration, publication, and publicity. The Bureau of Investigation was devoted to the study of the principles of homeopathy, the use of the repertory and materia medica, case-taking and record-keeping, and the preparation of drugs. The Bureau of Research and demonstration focused its attention on provings, the demonstration of *similia* in clinics and hospitals, laboratory research, and the correlation of homeopathy to chemistry, physics, electricity, psychology, sociology, and the other sciences. The Bureau of Publication reported on foundation activities, provided information for laypersons, reprinted relevant material that was out of print, maintained an index of homeopathic literature, and collected various memorabilia pertaining to homeopathy. Finally, the Bureau of Publicity devoted its efforts to supporting the laity with instruction in the fundamentals of homeopathy; encouraging laity to "think soundly and independently about medicine"; teaching them to take responsibility for their own health; coordinating visits and talks; establishing lay leagues; and supporting publicity. The magazine cost two dollars per year.[46]

The Homeopathic Survey, which ran for two years, was replaced by *The Layman's Weekly,* clear evidence of the growing partnership between physicians and laypersons in the homeopathic movement. Arthur B. Green (1884-1977), editor of the magazine, was a graduate of Harvard College (1907) and began his career as a civil engineer, designing factories, and making innovations for the pulp and paper industry. Along with his sister, Dr. Julia M. Green, he had been instrumental in establishing the AFH in Washington, DC, in 1924. He had also been lay editor of *The Homeopathic Survey.* Following the decision of the AFH to cut off funds for its publication due to opposition by medical doctors to lay involvement in what was perceived as strictly medical matters, Green wrote and mailed out a one-page weekly first titled *The Homeopathic Bulletin* (later called *The Layman's Bulletin*) for eighteen years without foundation funding. Circulation varied from 80 to 250. In 1941, Arthur Green became a trustee for the AFH and soon after became director of its Bureau of Laymen and, in 1947, editor of *The Layman Speaks,* intended as "an educational journal, a news journal, and an open layman's forum." The journal's name was suggested by Dr. Ray W. Spalding, chair of the board of trustees of the AFH. The magazine's circulation rose steadily from an initial 80 subscriptions to approximately 1,200 in the late 1960s. The magazine ran an annual deficit of more than $3,000 for the AFH, an amount that remained steady throughout its forty-one-year history.[47]

The intent of *The Layman Speaks* was severalfold. Recognizing that undergraduate teaching of homeopathy had not been successful and that postgraduate teaching offered the most promise for the future of the school, the editors intended that the articles be for the intelligent, thinking laity intent on seeking cures, if cures were possible, in a simple, effective, and safe manner. The individualization required for successful homeopathic prescribing required that the patient have some understanding of what the doctor was trying to do, how he or she accomplished it, and to what extent the patient must cooperate with the doctor in reporting symptoms and removing the obstacles to cure. This meant fighting specialism in medicine and countering public opinion formed by radio, magazines, and newspapers which demanded miracle drugs, histamines, vaccines, vitamins, and other products of the large pharmaceutical houses.[48] Bringing the truth of homeopathy to the layperson meant that fewer persons would be misled by the publicity behind the so-called miracle drugs and instead would understand the true laws on which medicine rested. In addition, the magazine was intent on preserving through publicity the right of adults to determine the form or manner of treatment or care for the cure or prevention of disease. "As time rolls on," wrote Arthur Green, "decisions of vast importance must be made on questions involving medical freedom. . . . If the lay public plays its full and proper part and plays it intelligently, democracy in America will once more be vindicated."[49] Finally, the magazine was intended to bring laypersons into active work on behalf of homeopathy. This included formal courses of instruction (called *Qualifying Course for Laymen*) with a qualified leader and designed to give the laity the principles of homeopathy and prepare them to make intelligent and correct selections of their doctors, and to cooperate intelligently with those doctors in the management of their health.[50]

Over its forty-one-year history, *The Layman Speaks* and its company of avid readers were the happy beneficiaries of Green's careful editorial hand. Nevertheless, there were problems with carrying out the lay education program. The "Qualifying Course for Laymen" consisted of fifteen weekly meetings using a syllabus formulated by the AFH and taught by a leader who was himself a layperson. Successful students received a certificate from the AFH. The fifteen topics were arranged as follows:

1. Medicine: as Distinct from Sanitation, Hygiene, Surgery
2. Object or Purpose of Medicine
3. Palliation, Suppression, Cure
4. Cure
5. What Is to Be Cured
6. Individualization
7. Case-Taking and the Law of Similars
8. Red Cross First Aid and Homeopathy
9. The Reason Why Medicine Must Be Internal
10. The Germ Theory
11. The Proving of Remedies
12. Potentization of Remedies
13. Homeopathy and the Modern Sciences
14. Homeopathy—Post-Graduate Medical Specialty
15. Preparation of the Homeopathic Physician

Critics felt that the "Qualifying Course for Laymen" and its examination misled the laity into concluding that they were qualifying to prescribe across-the-board remedies when, in actuality, they were being prepared to only administer first aid. Moreover, while lay groups helped to teach potential patients what to say in repertory symptomatology and what to expect, they were often accused of fostering self-medication. In addition, there was the issue of course readings. In Boston, the class studied Herbert A. Roberts' *Philosophy and Art of Cure by Homeopathy,* and James Tyler Kent's *Lectures on Homeopathic Philosophy,* neither of which was easy to read. In fact, both books were written with the graduate medical student in mind and much in them was viewed as beyond the capacity of the laity.[51]

Thus, the stakes were both real and burdensome for homeopathic physicians when they fostered the formation of lay groups. To be sure, the readership of *The Layman Speaks* found it sometimes difficult to discern the magazine's intent given the shrinking number of physicians who were able to treat the growing influx of patients. For some readers of the magazine, the issue became how much information was it possible to print for the laity without actually practicing medicine. For those who saw few physicians entering the ranks of homeopathy, it was important for the magazine to provide technical articles in order that the laity might better understand homeopathy and be able to care for the health situations with which they faced. The older generation of laity, however, found the magazine difficult to read due to their inability to understand medical case histories and their limited interest in the listing of various drugs used for treatment.

Upon Green's retirement in 1974, the National Center for Homeopathy assumed financial responsibility for the magazine. That same year, editorial responsibilities fell to Richard Dykeman and later to Alain Naudé. In 1976, Dykeman rattled the readership with an editorial announcing "disturbing reports" that had reached his office concerning attempts by the laity "to prescribe for themselves and others." While the administration of drugs for minor first-aid conditions was all well and good for the educated layperson, some had chosen to go beyond that threshold by "establishing a type of limited practice." This, Dykeman warned, would "do more harm to the future of Homeopathy than the good they are trying to do by filling the current lack of physicians."

> Homeopathy has been forced to the fringe of traditional medical practice by those whose motives are at best self-centered and at worse considered criminal. If the practice of Homeopathy degenerates to the hands of unlicensed laypersons, it will be playing into the hands of those who seek its total abolition. Even the layperson who suggests a remedy to a friend could theoretically be charged with practicing medicine in some states. Many dedicated Homeopaths are laboring to coalesce their scattered forces into a united movement that can achieve the goals we all seek. This cannot be accomplished if the actions of some, no matter how well intentioned, serve to undermine the constructive efforts now underway.[52]

When Alain Naudé of San Francisco, former editor and publisher of *Homeotherapy,* became editor of *The Layman Speaks* in 1977, he refused to endorse the practice of lay prescribing; however, he did not object to using the magazine's pages to stimulate discussion on the factors that made it necessary for laypersons to prescribe for themselves and others. This was the ultimate dilemma. If a homeopathic renaissance was going to occur, it appeared likely that it would take place on account of the laity's work and not because of any organized medical schools or the presence of trained homeopathic physicians. Yet, the growing number of laypersons who had begun to practice brought to question homeopathy's very status and future. If the laity were allowed to practice, would this create a legal difference between homeopathy and regular medicine? If so, did this imply a legal difference between the two, that is, that homeopathy was not a medicine in the same legal sense as regular medicine? If the laity dispensed with all credentials, standards, and controls, did they not became a law unto themselves? Equally so, would they not be equated with the fringe therapies of health food stores and the occult? Would homeopathic remedies, once recognized by the United States government on par with the pharmacopoeia of regular medicine, lose their status and be considered nonmedical therapy on the grounds that "holistic healthcare" was not medicine? The ramifications were obviously far reaching. With no recognized homeopathic qualifications, credentials, or standards remaining within the profession, only the establishment of new homeopathic schools offered any guarantee of competence. The alternative was "some paramedic role far below allopathy, and far removed from really sick patients." For Naudé, the proper role of the laity was bringing their energy, intelligence, and dedication together in an effort to establish homeopathic medical schools, thereby starting a movement that would give homeopathy "an incomparable new brilliance and power, such as to bedazzle even the giants of the past."[53]

The magazine ceased publication in 1978.

LUYTIES PHARMACAL COMPANY

When asked to speak before the convention of the AIH in 1968, Forrest Murphy, president of Luyties Pharmacal Company, accepted with enthusiasm. Committed to the doctrines of Hahnemann, he nonetheless expressed his puzzlement with the complacency of so many of its adherents. The threat to homeopathy's future, he argued, came not from the government, not from the AMA, but from the apathy and inertia evident among its own members. He came to the conclusion that only a "few truly dedicated lay people" were continuing to keep homeopathy alive. Murphy reported that he oversaw the liquidation of the William Luyties estate, whose Luyties Pharmacal Company had been in the homeopathic business since 1853.* He admitted to buying the entire business from the estate for about the price of the real estate alone. In effect, the homeopathic operation "was thrown in because no one wanted to buy it." Although Murphy had expected to liquidate the operation and retool the 36,000 square foot building for another business venture, he decided instead to study homeopathy with the idea of continuing with the company's line of products. "I decided that homeopathy was not dead, nor decadent, nor doomed, but rather neglected and mistreated by its own people, not by anyone on the outside, only by the homeopaths themselves."[54]

In his decision to reintroduce homeopathic remedies, Murphy chose to direct his revitalization at the laity because he found their responsiveness much greater than the professionals'. To achieve this objective, he prepared educational material for interested laypersons, sending out mailings on the Schüssler biochemic tissue salts and explaining similars, potencies, dilutions, and triturations that most simply took for granted. His next objective was to look at the export field, recognizing that homeopathy enjoyed a higher level of esteem in Asia. Finally, he decided to manufacture a wide range of potencies so that doctors and laity could order with a reasonable assurance of obtaining the requested potency. All of this resulted in increased sales and the satisfaction of affording genuine cure for the sick.[55]

Murphy noted that many people were already familiar with homeopathy, but unable to receive treatment because of decreasing numbers of homeopathically trained doctors. To correct this, Murphy urged the extension of home study courses for the laity. He also pointed out that European, American, and Asian homeopathies differed from each other and that these differences had to be respected. He explained:

> None are all right—none are all wrong—but you can be might sure that only a premise as sound and as irrefutable as Dr. Hahnemann's SIMILIA SIMILIBUS CURANTUR would

*The company was established by Dr. Herman Luyties who moved to St. Louis in 1850 and started a small retail pharmacy. During the period of westward expansion, Luyties became the main source of remedies for frontier families and their doctors. After his death in 1896, his son, August, expanded the business. In 1912, it moved to laboratories and offices at 4200 Laclede Avenue in the heart of the St. Louis medical district.

stand up and continue to flourish under as many versions, interpretations, and interpolations as we experience in world homeopathy.[56]

VULGARIZATION

In a presentation before the annual meeting of the AIH in 1968, Roger A. Schmidt, MD (d. 1975), former president of the AIH, reported that homeopathy had reached its acme under the guiding leadership of James T. Kent, but that it was now time to end its separateness and become an integral part of the field of medicine. Homeopathy's past sectarianism was no longer desirable or necessary. This position, Schmidt admitted, went against the desire of the laity to advocate "a complete, unique system of medicine." But while the laity's position had been shared by the profession for many decades, it had alienated mainstream medicine with its partisan point of view. Commending the AFH for its publication of *The Layman Speaks,* he noted, however, that the magazine was not supported by the homeopathic profession because of its hostility to conventional medicine. "The old time polemics of accusing and vilifying our opponents" had proved ineffective and contrary to the AIH's hope for eventual integration into modern medicine. Even more serious, Schmidt was troubled by the laity's "vulgarization" of homeopathy. In their persistent and often unschooled efforts to advance the cause of their sectarian philosophy, the laity too often stood apart from the ranks of professionals. For Schmidt, the future of homeopathy lay in the recruitment of academically trained physicians from Europe, the East, and South America, not from expanding the role of the laity. The future lay in newly trained professionals rather than from the thorny vulgarizations advocated by laypersons.[57]

In 1977, the *JAIH* noted a "painful conflict" emerging within the homeopathic world, a disagreement over policy that had become as serious and as divisive as any of the previous doctrinal differences that had plagued homeopathy in the past. This new conflict concerned the growing number of laypersons who had begun practicing in the absence of trained professionals. The journal questioned whether these activities, if allowed to continue, would force legal barriers between homeopathy and regular medicine. If homeopathy was determined *not* to be a medicine, then what was it? The question struck at the very definition of homeopathy itself.[58]

From the prospective of the AIH, the decline in numbers of trained homeopathic physicians had been offset by a virtual explosion of lay practitioners, most of whom had practiced domestic homeopathy on themselves and their families and then gradually extended their healing skills to other households before moving into general practice. This was patently wrong. "People who dispense with all credentials, standards, and controls become a law unto themselves, and need fulfill no requirements beyond those of their own integrity, conscience, and understanding," wrote the editor of the *JAIH.* Even if lay prescribers were highly motivated, they could not possibly fulfill those standards without some degree of medical training. This had been repeatedly enunciated by Hahnemann, Constantine Hering, J. T. Kent, Elizabeth Wright Hubbard, and others through the decades. Homeopathy practiced by laypersons had no accountability. In its new robes, it became "fringe therapy" with kits of domestic remedies sold through health stores and occult bookshops. In this mode, homeopathy became "misunderstood, distorted, dishonored, exploited."[59]

In 1978, the AIH called for its members to "take stock" of its position and to formulate a policy for the future. Given the decline of professional homeopathy and the "uncontrollable wave of irresponsible homeopathic activity outside the profession," the AIH had the challenge of defining its purpose and reason for existence.

> Is it only a professional fraternity whose members communicate among themselves and share experience, monitor internal conformity to the professional and ethical rules of the guild, admit, or refuse candidates who want to join the group? Or is it the entity to which the destiny of homeopathy in this country has been entrusted, so that it must defend homeopathy itself—its principles, its political and social survival, its professional integrity? In the first instance we have concern merely with the domestic matters of a group; in the second we have allegiance to something great and important beyond this group, and duty, and a mission. Actually the AIH must fulfill both these functions, and they are not contradictory. It is responsible to the corps of homeopathic physicians in the United States, and beyond and above

> that, to Homeopathy itself, to the tradition and the potential bequeathed by the great homeopaths of the past.

For the editor, the only school of homeopathy which could lay claim to the name was the homeopathy of Hahnemann. Anything less was unacceptable. Equally important, homeopathy had to abandon all efforts to present itself in terms acceptable to regular medicine. This is because the thought, categories, and philosophy of allopathy were contrary to the principles of homeopathy. True homeopaths must "rediscover" the principles of Hahnemann—principles that could not be divorced from the broader spiritual realm from which they originated. "Homeopathy is the medical expression of a spiritual and vitalistic understanding of man," explained the editor. "If we divorce the two, Homeopathy will wither like a plant without roots." To achieve this, American homeopaths had to align themselves with professional homeopaths in other countries and work with them to formulate common doctrines and goals. If this was not done, American homeopathy would be forced into "inviting the laymen to start schools in which Homeopathy will be removed from the profession forever."[60]

Chapter 4

Postwar Trends

At the close of the Second World War, homeopaths at home and abroad sought to reestablish contacts interrupted by the war and to resume their collective and cooperative efforts. At the first postwar meeting of the Council of the International Homeopathic League which met in London in 1947, William Gutman, MD, of New York proposed the establishment of an International Homeopathic Research Council as an instrument for future research initiatives. The institute's functions were to include the proving of drugs; the collection of toxicological facts; the collection of pharmacological data which confirmed the Law of Similia; the publication of case histories; the pooling and comparing of statistical information; clinical trials of both old and new remedies; publishing abstracts reviewing international homeopathic literature; identifying laboratory experiments that approach homeopathy through modern physics; the preparation of homeopathic remedies; the incorporation of information for repertories; encouraging scientific cooperation; and the publication of an international homeopathic bulletin.[1]

For Robert H. Farley, MD, writing in 1948, the pressing need for homeopathy was to identify research programs and pursue them with vigor. While nonhomeopathic topics might be interesting, only those research topics with the potential for furthering the purposes of homeopathy were given the highest priority. This meant the continued development of remedies by provings; republication of the standard homeopathic texts; publication of new works on homeopathic problems; collecting clinically confirmed symptoms; better indexing of repertories; improvement of the punch card repertory project; and follow up on cases reported cured or helped. In laboratory research, tasks included measuring the effects of drugs upon diseased organisms; exploring the degree that a similar drug may influence susceptibility, immunity, idiosyncrasy, allergy, and anaphylaxis; identifying the minimum effective dose; and exploring the effects of dilution, trituration, succussion, age of preparation, light, and heat upon the minimum effective preparation.[2]

Now that instruments existed to measure the energy of potentized remedies, homeopaths felt an awakened sense of importance and hoped to counter the humiliation they had faced in previous decades. Not only had the Baruch Committee on Physical Medicine (1944-51), financed by industrialist Bernard M. Baruch and headed by Dr. Ray Lyman Wilbur, declared that drugs were becoming obsolete, but homeopathic remedies were also being admitted to the official French Codex and the homeopathic movement was growing in India, Pakistan, and countries in South America. In England, by act of Parliament, homeopathic hospitals were authorized to maintain their independent specialties. In France, homeopaths were pleased to claim Pierre Curie, director of the Curie Institute for Radiology, as a homeopathic physician. For many of homeopathy's advocates, Hahnemann's concept of dynamization, interpreted in the light of modern physics, suggested that the electric energy present in potentized remedies was the force that ultimately met the disease and destroyed it.[3]

ATOMIC ENERGY

In spite of initial skepticism voiced in the editorials of the *JAIH,* the possibility of a relationship between atomic energy and the remedial power of potentized medicines ignited a firestorm of discussion among professional and lay homeopaths in the years following the Second World War. To rank-and-file members in the AIH, there appeared to be no proof that drug atoms were "smashed" by either the succussion or trituration processes, there being insufficient power in the shaking or in the heaviest mortar and pestle to achieve that capability. The fact remained, however, that highly dilute remedies had "an astonishing degree of curative energy" and how this happened remained a paradox and was "at present impossible of explanation." It was a fact of nature "which we have to accept but cannot understand or elucidate," explained the editor. That being said, the AIH as an organization refused to support speculation that the atomic bomb provided "a tenable theory to account for the action of homeopathic remedies."[4]

On the other hand, individual homeopaths took an entirely different approach. K. C. Hiteshi, MD, insisted that the development of the atomic bomb verified the law of dynamization "beyond all doubt." It was nothing less than the "disassociation of matter" that converted massive energy by means of triturating, diluting, or by some other chemical process into infinitesimals as laid down in homeopathic practice.[5] Similarly, William P. Mowry, MD, of Michigan noted two types of atomic energy: one which occurred when the mass and energy system of an atom split into protons, electrons, and neutrons; and another when the energy inherent in the atom formed a single drug molecule. Focusing his attention on the latter, he explained that the single potentized drug was "far more powerful in its purely medicinal action than the mass or physical dosage of the same drug." In the transformation from the physical form to the pure energy form, the drug changed from its inert form into "self-moving, live, penetrating energy."[6] Once transformed, "pure energy" drugs would not harm healthy tissues, only the diseased part of the organism, and would restore the patient's recuperative powers. For a pure energy drug to work, it had to be administered by a properly trained doctor, nurse, or assistant. Mowry's analysis was enough to convince Fred B. Morgan, president of the AIH in 1947, to recommend further research into the fundamentals of homeotherapeutics and to remark that "there is enough atomic energy in the small dose to set diseased, disarranged life forces operating in a healthful orderly manner."[7]

From the perspective of numerous homeopaths, the age of atomic energy offered great promise to the treatment of disease. "The science of physics, the release of power contained in the atom and the import of vibrations and frequencies no longer make it illogical or difficult to accept the action of high potencies in their role of restoring order in a deranged vital organism," explained Arthur H. Grimmer (1874-1967) of Chicago, a pupil of Kent and president of the AIH in 1953. Today's science was now verifying truths announced more than a century earlier by Hahnemann.[8]

During the 1950s, Dr. Amaro Azevedo of Brazil advanced the proposition that atomic energy was the starting point in understanding the action of homeopathic remedies in the organism. Its action had been foreseen by Hahnemann when he developed his system of dynamization. In homeopathic dynamizations, one encountered curative substances that were highly diluted and therefore incapable of any significant chemical reaction. For Azevedo, an actual "fission" occurred when the medicine was dynamized. With these remarks, high dilutions once again came into fashion. Besides the well-known 30X potency, now there were references to even higher potencies labeled 10M, 50M, and CM. In the United States, laboratories making 1 to 30th dilutions employed the Hahnemannian method while potencies between 30 and 1,000 utilized the hand-made Korsakov method, and for dilutions above 1,000, dynamizers used the Thomas Skinner (1825-1906) or Kentian methods. In France, the high potencies were prepared according to Korsakov's method and in England by the Hahnemannian method. In Brazil, Argentina, Mexico, and Chile, laboratories preferred the use of turbo-dynamizers to make their medicines.[9]

Generally, homeopaths were willing to affirm that the roots of atomic energy could be found in Hahnemann's drug potentization theory. Just as the atom when split by bombardment freed protons, electrons, and neutrons that escaped with tremendous force and energy, so also the homeopathic drug when properly potentized, "goes down deep into the body, mind and spirit annihilating the most latent disease from the physique, the mind and spirit of the diseased person," explained Dr. J. D. Vaishnav in 1968.[10]

Along with the renewed popularity of the higher potencies came interest in devices such as the Geiger counter and scintillation counter for tracing minute amounts of matter and observing physiological and biochemical reactions. Advocates of high-dilution therapy trusted that radioautography (a technique used to locate a radioactive substance) would reveal what had heretofore been only conjectural as to the maximal effects of their potencies. Now with the use of radioactive tracer materials homeopaths thought it possible to observe the action of minute amounts of drug on the body.[11]

In a paper before a meeting of the Southern Homeopathic Medical Association in 1955, Mary I. Senseman, MD, added to the discussion of fission by speculating that the source of a potentized drug's effect on an organism was due to the formation of an electrical circuit within the body of the physician at the time of succussion and the transference of that energy to the sick patient.

> Treatment of disease by the use of homeopathic remedies may be compared in some ways to the continuing fission which is instrumental in what is commonly called chain reaction. If, in a mass of fissionable material, a single neutron is captured by one atom of this material, the atom splits, releasing at that time more than one neutron. One of these may be captured, causing a second fission or split, and the same process can continue. The end effect will be a continuing release of energy. We may draw a comparison with a much more complex process, the action of a correct remedy. Let us assume that our mass of fissionable material is an individual—an ill body. Now assume that our neutron (one of correct energy to have a high probability of fission) is a homeopathic remedy—the correct remedy of the right potency. That remedy causes the start of a series of reactions in the ill body, which also releases energy, the end result being a correction toward the normal of the deviated metabolic pathway which was typified by the illness. The cure has not depended upon mass of dose (number of neutrons initially given); it has not depended on relief or suppression of one symptom (one fission); but it has depended on the right remedy at the right time in the right potency.[12]

In order to understand the rules governing high- and low-potency medicines, Horace E. Reed, MD, of Dover, Ohio, a member of the AIH board of directors in 1954, explained that the true homeotherapeutist began with the knowledge that every substance in nature was endowed with energy. "This energy is the force which binds the atoms of that substance into a molecule"; and since no two substances were identical, neither were their energies. Through the processes of dilution and succussion, the energy that the substance contained was released, allowing the freed energy to enter the sick constitution and bring relief. Low-potency remedies gave off little energy when they entered the sick constitution and therefore required frequent repetition. By contrast, the higher potencies (now called "high energy" medicines) released greater amounts of energy and required fewer repetitions.[13] By the 1960s, a compromise had been reached between the low- and high-potency advocates, whereby all potencies had their rightful place in homeopathic practice. In the compromise, homeopaths chose the following rules: the use of low potencies, from the tincture to 6X in gross pathological conditions; medium potencies from 6X to the 200th in functional disorders; and high potencies from the 200th and up in mental states, psychosomatic, or chronic conditions without gross pathology.[14]

With the expanded use of Nuclear Magnetic Resonance (NMR) instrumentation in medical research in the late 1960s, biochemists and physicists looked for signs of molecular change when specific substances interacted with body proteins. For homeopaths, NMR gave promise of showing changes caused by the higher potencies where the medicine was beyond the molecular level of testing.[15] In time, it was hoped that modern quantum mechanics and spectral theory would provide additional answers to the perturbations of health produced by the provings of drugs, the restoration of health produced by the selected similimum, and the structural patterns brought to the eye through electromagnetic spectrum.

With advances in physics, homeopaths sought newer ways to explain how their potencies worked. "We are told by the savants of physics that matter and energy are interchangeable under varying conditions," explained Arthur H. Grimmer, MD, "and that both are characterized by their specific rates of vibration; in fine all matter from its crudest to its finest form and expression is vibratory in nature." With the understanding that energy or force of all types was simply matter "transformed to higher rates of vibration," he concluded that homeopaths had found the secret to the power of their potencies. Simply put, "potencies consist[ed] of matter raised to extremely high rates of vibration simulating the quality and vibratory rate of the life force that animates the human body." According to Grimmer, these forces were not only vibratory but also had a "directional flow" or "polarity."

> Thus we see that the finest grain of sand made up primarily of tiny electrons and the mightiest sun whirling in space are both governed by the same mysterious but mighty inexorable force, that force emanating from God whose guiding omnipotent intelligence holds and binds the fabric of the cosmos in perfect unity

> and order. This universal law of electromagnetic polarity performs an important role in homeopathics. The remedies of our Materia Medica are classified into four groups according to their polarity, viz.: negative, positive, neutral and bi-polar, and the blood of all patients will come in one of these four groups. The individual whose blood test is negative with an intensity measuring 12 ohm in electrical resistance will be found to be at least in approximately good health, or under the influence of the similimum will give the normal negative polarity reading as long as the remedy continues to act. The similimum will restore all abnormal polarities to the normal with an abatement of all adverse symptoms and improved health in the whole clinical picture as long as the remedy holds and acts.[16]

Discussions in the 1950s suggested that the energy forces within the cell as well as forces outside of it posed areas of important research in the healing arts. This included thought waves whose frequencies operated similar to those of the heavy metals when highly diluted. Considering how easy the thought wave of the sick could be influenced for better or worse by the physician, Allen C. Neiswander, associate editor for the *JAIH,* urged homeopaths to weigh equally the state of the mind and mental symptoms in studying the patient.[17]

EASTERN PHILOSOPHY

As homeopaths entered the 1960s and the so-called Age of Aquarius, they found it less necessary to explain the curative process of their dematerialized medicines using the dominant biomedical paradigm of molecular reductionism. As noted earlier, the research of radiologist Dr. William Ernest Boyd in the 1920s at Glasgow Homeopathic Hospital was credited with confirming the active principle of medicines potentized beyond the Avogadro limit.* However, his "emanometer" experiments, undertaken to demonstrate vital bioenergetic properties, were quickly debunked by a procession of biomedical scientists who rejected any inclination to consider "immaterial energies," especially when steeped in the "dynamic notions of vitalism." Faced with this conundrum, homeopaths chose to reconceptualize their dynamic,

---

*A dilution beyond 1×10^{-24}.

holistic, and vitalistic concepts of health and healing by seeking solace in Eastern medical traditions.[18]

By the late 1950s and early 1960s, homeopathy was forging ahead in the British Isles, in India, and in Central America, Mexico, and Brazil. In the United States, postgraduate courses of six-week duration were being offered using faculty from India, Switzerland, Barbados, Argentina, and Mexico. The AIH began publishing an increasing number of articles written by Indian homeopaths and drawing yogic vision into the discussion of Hahnemann's insight. Viewing the human organism as a triune organization, Dr. B. K. Sarkar of Calcutta wrote of the life and mind, with the soul, or Jivatman as the substratum. Man was an infinitely composite being, "a bundle or dynamo of energy and this energy is nothing but the force of consciousness." Borrowing freely from the writings of Sri Aurobindo and Sri Anilbaran Roy, he attempted to show the metaphysical implications behind psora and the idea of dynamization. There was a direct correlation between the metaphysical ideas of Hahnemann and those of Eastern philosophy.[19] For Sarkar, the principles of homeopathy sprang from "phenomenologic, visualizing, intuitive, analogizing thought" as opposed to "causal, conceptual and discursive thought." Thus, Hahnemann's ideas were in accord with the advanced beliefs of Albert Einstein, Max Plank, and others who had sought "to do away with the notion of causality altogether."[20]

In place of Western science's reductionistic mechanisms, homeopaths increasingly turned to Eastern concepts of life, death, sickness, and health. In part, the catalyst for this had been the earlier interest in physics which broadened homeopathic research into a more sophisticated set of concepts that went beyond conventional science. These, in turn, led to a concept of the body that was not confined to the physical form alone. The body was now viewed as a three-layered system: *physical, etheric,* and *aura.* The physical side was the core of the body, electrical in origin. By that was meant the brain generated electricity through the action of water and the metallic compounds coursing through it. The body also generated a magnetic field that was known as the etheric layer which vibrated rapidly and extended about an eighth of an inch to six inches from the body and represented the degree of an individual's vitality. The depth of this etheric layer fluctuated with the body's health. Beyond the etheric layer was the aura whose origin was electromagnetic and thought of as the "soul" or "oversoul" of the organism. It was the ultimate purification of this level which permitted the merging or "unification with the Divine."[21]

The concepts behind homeopathy fit well with ancient Indian medicine and with its belief in the efficacy of immaterial entities. No longer was it a struggle to conceptualize homeopathic potencies. Inspired by the writings of Hahnemann and Kent, potencies prepared by succussion were accepted easily by Indian healers. Nor did the fear of science trouble these healers. "No microscope, however powerful, will reveal the spirit of any substance," wrote Dr. A. V. Subramanian. Homeopathic potencies could not be perceived by any instrument whatsoever in a physical plane. In spite of this, the Indian philosophy defined as God or Brahman the universal spirit that pervaded everything in the universe, movable or immovable, seen or unseen. Vital force in homeopathic parlance was the "sukshuma sariram" of Indian philosophy. When Kent explained that medicine could not be divorced from theology, his concept was but a reflection of the Upanishadic aphorism: "From Him who is whole has issued all this whole."[22]

Tarig Kuraishy, a pharmacist and president of the Health Research Institute in Las Vegas specializing in the manufacture of homeopathic medicines, commended modern science for "waking up" to the existence of this supernatural phenomenon and showing a willingness to accept unconventional explanations to explain the vital force. Concepts such as field theory, quantum theory, and the relativity theory heralded a new era, voiding the conventional norms of past science. In this new paradigm, mental and spiritual conditions along with matter and energy were interchangeable, enabling a person "to revert from the physical to the etheric and back again." Levitation, the bending of metallic objects with thought, and the violation of Newtonian physics and gravitational forces were all part of Kuraishy's field of vision and had an application to homeopathy, particularly in explaining potentization which continued to be misunderstood in chemical or materialistic terms. Admitting that ascending the potency ladder and the steady exponential decrease in any measurable drug substance were concepts unimaginable to reductionist medicine, Kuraishy viewed them as perfectly understandable by virtue of an increase in the electromagnetic field. As he explained, the potentization process released particles called "deltrons" from the molecules in solution and these, in turn, interacted with the etheric level. With each additional succussion/trituration, more deltrons were detached to increase the etheric activity. Although allopathy was limited in its ability to explain the action of drug substances in the human organism, this was not the case with Eastern philosophy (Yogi) which used psycho-energetic phenomenon, and the physical/etheric levels of the organism to understand illness. Other therapeutic approaches could also directly affect the etheric plane. These included the laying-on-of-hands by which individuals developed a "third eye" to see the aura and diagnose man's illnesses and serving as channels of universal energies to affect the electrodynamic field; and acupuncture which connected the vital organs to the body's energy circuits.[23]

GEORGE VITHOULKAS

In 1974, the Greek civil engineer George Vithoulkas (b. 1932) was "discovered" by Dr. Maesimund P. Panos (B. 1912), chair of the trustees of the AFH, at a meeting of the International Homeopathic League (Liga) in Athens, Greece. Soon, he became spokesman for a new generation of homeopaths including Bill Gray, David Wember, Nick Nossaman, Dean Crothers, Richard Mosikowitz, Karl Robinson, and Sandra M. Chase.[24] Like Kent before him, Vithoulkas was a high-potency advocate whose seminars at the Pacific College of Naturopathic Medicine focused on symptoms of the mind, the emotions, and the psychological approach in general. The director of education at the Hahnemann Medical Clinic in Berkeley, California, Vithoulkas was also author of *Homeopathy, Medicine of the New Man* (1971) the textbook, *The Science of Homeopathy* (1978), and *A New Model of Health and Disease* (1991). He was also founder of the Athenian School of Homeopathic Medicine and cofounder of the International Foundation for Homeopathy located in Seattle, Washington, which closed in 1998.

Vithoulkas held that the substantive differences existing between homeopathic and conventional medicines were grounded in subjective versus objective or reductionist concepts of matter and energy. Starting with this assertion, he deduced that homeopathy dealt with the mental and emotional level of the individual patient and, as such, operated in a multidimensional energy-chain that existed outside the laboratory-based quantitative sciences. Homeopathy, a system of therapy based on stimulating the energy level of the individual, reached out to the patient through energized remedies that operated on the electromagnetic level of the physical body. It was a medicine unlike any other in its visionary promise and in its possibilities; indeed, it stood on the threshold of transforming mankind into a more highly spiritualized being.[25]

In his *The Science of Homeopathy,* published in 1980, Vithoulkas sought to restate the principles of health and disease in "a comprehensive rational system" that could be clinically verified. To accomplish this, he began by viewing individuals in their totality, that is, understanding the individual as a functioning conscious being within the universe, the solar system, the nation, the immediate society, the geographical location, and family. Since it was always the whole person, either actively or passively, that performed a particular function, he considered it profoundly important to discern the individual in an integrated manner rather than the molecular, organ, or psychological levels alone. Although he stressed the importance of the integrated whole, he evaluated health and disease from the perspective of three levels or hierarchies: the mental or spiritual plane which registered changes in understanding or consciousness; the emotional or psychic level which registered the range of states such as love or hatred, joy or sadness; and the physical plane which registered the gradations of the body in terms of its organs and systems. While signs of health or disease registered in each of the three levels of existence, all three worked as a totality.[26]

Drawing from both ancient and modern writers, Vithoulkas held that, unlike the materialist view which explained life in mechanical terms, a vital force or energy directed the life of the organism and connected it with the "ultimate Unity of the universe." As the spokesman for modern homeopathy, however, he chose to emphasize the scientific and less mysterious side of homeopathy by substituting the ideas of systems theorist Fritjof Capra, author of *The Tao of Physics* (1975), and the concepts of theoretical physicist Albert Einstein (1879-1955) for Kent's Swedenborgianism. With a more modern understanding of this ancient concept now possible through advances in physics in field theory, quantum theory, and relativity theory, he proceeded to assert the existence of a correlation between the three levels of existence and the electromagnetic field emanating from the individual in health and disease. The use of Kirlian photography and of Einstein's field theories were more complete descriptions of what Hahnemann and other homeopaths had postulated a hundred years earlier in their description of the qualities of the vital force.[27]

This led Vithoulkas to assert that an intelligent vital force animated the individual organism and behaved in the manner analogous to an electromagnetic field. This allowed the physician the opportunity to transform therapeutics into a form of energy medicine. Viewing the world at the atomic and subatomic levels where each substance or particle had a distinguishing electromagnetic wave, vibration, or frequency, he explained that, depending on the strength of a given stimulus, the organism responded and adjusted with visible effects on the mental, emotional, or physical levels. Although the organism's vital energy could manage most morbific stimuli, those that were stronger than the organism's defense mechanisms resulted in a change in the wave or vibration rate of the organism and a corresponding change in health. By finding a curative substance whose vibratory rate matched the frequency of susceptibility, the physician was able to disrupt the resulting deterioration of health and return the organism's defense mechanisms to their proper level.[28]

In seeking the therapy most apt to strengthen the organism's defensive mechanisms, Vithoulkas spoke of three possibilities: acupuncture, laying-on-of-hands, and the use of the homeopathic potentized remedy. Although the first two were highly effective, there were too few masters of acupuncture and far too few individuals who were "spiritually evolved" enough to effectively channel their energies to solving health problems. This left homeopathic science which, building on the insight afforded by Hahnemann's Law of Similia and the symptom-complex, brought together the vibrational level of a particular therapeutic substance with that of the patient's defense mechanisms. Using the principle of resonance between the therapeutic agent and the vibration level of the organism, Vithoulkas potentized specific substances to stimulate the electromagnetic plane of the organism. By increasing the energy capacity of a substance through succussion or trituration, the homeopath was able to direct the substance's energy level using the Law of Similia to the organism, enhancing its vitality and thereby returning the organism to its original state. Once the correct potency was reached, the organism's response brought about the disappearance of symptoms. Vithoulkas also claimed that potencies beyond Avogadro's number had proven successful. While there was no current explanation for this phenomenon, he insisted that sufficient energy was released by the succussion or trituration processes that even when the original substance was no longer present, "the remaining energy in the solvent can be continually enhanced ad infinitum." The therapeutic energy still retained the "vibrational frequency" of the original substance, explained Vithoulkas, "but the energy has been enhanced to such a degree that it is capable of stimulating the dynamic plane of the patient sufficiently to produce a cure."[29]

Critical to the correct treatment of patients using homeopathic theory was the mastering of its tools—plant, mineral, animal, and diseased products—which came from a variety of sources and which required an accurate recording of their manifestations on a healthy individual before matching them to the symptom-picture (resonant frequencies) of the patient. This required an accurate reading of both the primary and secondary effects of a potentized substance on all three levels of the organism (mental, emotional, and physical) in the hours, days, and even months following its administration on a healthy body. Only when the vibration rate of the sick patient matched exactly with the vibration rate of the potentized substance did the patient experience a lasting alleviation of symptoms. Given the totality of the symptom-complex, it was possible to identify or know each remedy by its particular "form," "shape," "personality," "soul," or "essence." In other words, the remedy's "resonant frequency" produced a symptom image which the homeopath then sought to match with the patient's symptom-picture. Vithoulkas believed that Kent's *Lectures on Homeopathic Materia Medica with New Remedies* (1905) provided the best compilation of remedy "essences" or "personalities."[30]

Vithoulkas did not go unchallenged. Jost Kunzli von Fimelsberg, MD, author of *Kent's Repertorium Generale* (1987), was critical of Vithoulkas's approach and felt that his students were "trying hard to analyze the mentals, and the emotional aspects of the patient as though they were qualified psychologists." He chided Vithoulkas for leading his disciples into a "psychological labyrinth" from which there were few escapes.[31] Kunzli disliked as well Vithoulkas's overemphasis on the emotional level of the patient, giving each remedy an "essence," that is, such as identifying "cowardice" as the essence or symptomatology for lycopodium. This was dangerous path once embarked and had been opposed decades earlier by Constantine Hering as leading to the decline of homeopathy. Kunzli viewed the emphasis on essences among Vithoulkas's supporters as symptomatic of the efforts of young people "groping for stability, and trying to find it in an alien far Eastern religion and drugs."[32] Another critic, George A. Guess, MD, feared that too many homeopathic students, having only a superficial understanding of Vithoulkas's concepts, would gravitate exclusively to the "essences" and ignore other vital aspects of case analysis.[33]

However, these objections were not shared by all. Alan Levine, MD, of Madison, Wisconsin, took issue with Vithoulkas's critics. Having been trained in family medicine and psychiatry, and trained as well by Vithoulkas in a program established under the auspices of the International Foundation for Homeopathy, Levine argued that for the first time in decades classical homeopathy was "beginning to jump to life." He agreed with Kunzli that it would be good if homeopathy were taught as a specialty in medical schools, but doubted this would occur until enough individuals were trained in classical homeopathy to convince the skeptics of its validity.[34]

The Hahnemann Medical Clinic which opened in Berkeley had eleven practitioners, all trained by Vithoulkas and the International Foundation of Homeopathy. Based on a purely classical orientation, the clinic represented an important step in the re-establishment of homeopathic medical education. The purpose of the clinic was sixfold:

1. provide patients with classical homeopathic treatment;
2. create a program of courses in classical homeopathy;
3. educate the lay public in acute and first-aid prescribing;
4. create a full-time homeopathic medical school with full accreditation;
5. integrate licensed homeopathic pharmacy into the clinic;
6. conduct research proving the effectiveness of homeopathy.[35]

The growing interest in classical Kentian methods of homeopathy was due in large measure to the teachings of Vithoulkas and Bill Gray (b. 1942), a graduate of Stanford Medical School in 1970. Kentianism (i.e., the use of the single remedy given once in high potency) was the method of practice taught by the AFH in the 1950s and continued as the method of choice into the 1980s by the National Center for Instruction under the National Center for Homeopathy. Dr. Francisco Xavier Eizayaga of Buenos Aires taught a variation of this classical approach, advising the use of lower potencies for acute conditions, a technique taught earlier by Drs. Elizabeth Wright Hubbard and Allen Sutherland at the National Center for Instruction.[36]

PSYCHOSOMATIC MEDICINE

As homeopaths stretched their imaginations to encompass the breadth of the doctor-patient relationship, they began to show increased interest in psychosomatic medicine. By the 1950s, there appeared a number of articles recommending psychotherapy as a form of homeopathic treatment. The essential psychotherapeutic technique involved supportive treatment, suggestion, persuasion, ventilation, abreaction, and interpretation. By ventilation and abreaction was meant that the patient was encouraged to express his emotions freely, with the physician interrupting as little as possible.[37] William P. Britsch, Jr., who was neither a high- nor low-potency advocate, and who regretted the schism between the warring parties of similia and contraria, predicted that cellular pathology would eventually be replaced by a more widely accepted system of psychosomatic medicine.[38] Attributing the origination of psychosomatic medicine with Hahnemann who pleaded for more humane treatment of the insane, Britsch explained that the very nature of man proceeded from the spiritual and mental to the physical. For that reason, it was important to give due consideration to his mental and emotional symptoms. Along with diseases such as cancer, heart and kidney disease, patients also suffered from shock, frustration, anger, grief, and fear—all of which caused changes in the blood chemistry that resulted in pathological changes in the cell formation of the organism. Since the provings of the homeopath's remedies were rich in "perverted and abnormal mental states," it was essential to take into consideration medicines in their attenuated form to counter the aberrations.[39]

Owing to homeopathy's stance as representing something fundamentally different from allopathic medicine, the question most frequently asked by practitioners and patients alike was whether homeopathy had a greater affinity to spirituality. Given George Vithoulkas' definition of health as "freedom . . . from pain in the physical body . . . freedom from passion on the emotional level . . . and freedom from selfishness in the mental sphere," it seemed to Paul Bahder, MD, that homeopathy should be understood as a process of releasing the patient from the material level of disease and opening up health to the spiritual realm. In homeopathy, there was "no such thing as an objective interaction with the patient"; rather, homeopathy's relationship to the patient was at the level of "harmony, wisdom, love and transcendent stillness." Healing was not about removing or fighting a disease but of "coming to a greater level of health." This involved the soul of the patient and the very sanctity of life. It was this insight of focusing on the level of vital force that gave patients and practitioners the sense that homeopathy was something spiritual in nature and indeed reached beyond the soul to the "Spirit of the Universe." Nevertheless, Bahder felt there was a difference between homeopathy and spiritual healing. In effect, homeopathy was a transitional form of healing, at the juncture "between the conventional, mechanistic, chemical understanding of life, and the spiritual." Spiritual healing was when the patient submitted himself to God or the Spirit and where healing became more of a "gift" for finding spiritual peace with God. Homeopathy approached healing spiritually by not seeing disease as a physical phenomenon but as "an attribute of perception." It thus raised illness from a material sense "to a derangement of perception."[40]

Bernardo A. Merizalde, MD, postulated that homeopathy not only helped individuals pursue better health, but also introduced psychotherapeutic techniques that helped to restore the individual to higher spiritual and human virtues. Early evidence of this was found in Hahnemann's use of mesmerism, hydrotherapy, and massage modalities to accomplish a transformation from material to spiritual levels. This was the same transformation that had been the basis of historical alchemy as well as the objective of the Swiss psychoanalyst Carl G. Jung in the development of personality through psychotherapy.[41]

By the end of the twentieth century, the homeopathic lexicon had acquired new identifying terminology including "quantum medicine," "energy medicine," "complementary medicine," and "vibratory medicine"—despite the fact that homeopaths were unclear as to the actual meaning of the terms. Along with these identifiers came a plethora of new healing systems: Anthroposophical Medicine, Ayurvedic Medicine, Tibetan Medicine, Acupuncture, Herbal Medicine, Chiropractic, Naturopathy, Reiki, Alexander Technique, Craniosacral Therapy, Craniosacral-Visceral Therapy, Oki-Do, Reflexology, Deep Emotional Release Bodywork, Shiatsu, Rolfing, Light Ray Rejuvenation System, Aromatherapy, Essential Therapy, Healing Light, Jin Shin Do, Crystal Healing, Body Centered Psychotherapy, Psychodynamic Psychotherapy, Synergy Hypnosis, Past-Life Regression, Chi Therapy, Organic Process Therapy, Intuitive Psychotherapy, Soul Work, Neurolinguistic Programming, and Ericksonian Hypnosis. While many of these approaches claimed to be compatible with homeopathy, their actual relationship to the Law of Similia was tenuous at best. Few made any attempt to individualize treatment. In this new age of medicine, complained Domenick J. Masiello, the lines between and among alternative modalities blurred. There had been the "Hollywoodization" of health and, in the banality of that phenomenon, homeopathy fared no better than any of the other systems. Almost anything considered alternative was thought to connect to "holistic," "natural," and even "homeopathic." In a sense, the words designating alternative medical approaches had lost their individualistic meaning as print and broadcast media markets bunched them together to satisfy market forces.[42]

Along with quantum chemistry and solid state physics, writers in the 1990s turned to chaos theory as a means of explaining complex systems and understanding the modus operandi of homeopathy. In this new language, the sense of "order" was removed from the definition of healthy because it represented stasis. The term "chaos," on the other hand, no longer became a synonym for disorder but likened to fractals, a nonlinear concept that demonstrated "very definite, describable boundaries." In this new world, the vital force of Hahnemann became a subtle energy that could not "be predicted from the properties of the component parts." Using complexity theory, chaos theory, and systems theory resulted in dynamic changes in the nonlinear complex system of the patient, wherein health became an "emergent property" of the organic whole.[43]

The introduction of chaos theory stimulated great interest among homeopaths who saw the irregular, unpredictable behavior of natural phenomena as having relevance to the understanding of how certain perturbations such as energy medicine worked in stabilizing a system.

Homeopaths preferred a dynamic model that allowed for deductions to be made on the behavior of the whole organism rather than a reductionist view of the organism. By constructing a pattern of signs and symptoms from every part of the patient's mind and body, and including information that did not seem to fit any pattern, homeopaths concluded that these complex pictures actually followed a symptom-pattern of remedies derived from provings. Thus, the age-old practice of identifying very unique, rare, and strange symptoms actually pointed to a desired result.[44]

NEW CHALLENGES

Beginning in the 1980s, the hegemony of mechanistic and materialistic science faced renewed challenges from homeopathy. Prior to this time, homeopaths had generally played down the scientific side of their medicine hoping to avoid confrontation with the prestige of biomedicine's power base. In 1986, a controlled trial of homeopathic potency with pollen was conducted at the Glasgow Homeopathic Hospital and followed by other studies documenting the effectiveness of homeopathic medicines potentized to the point where, at least in theory, none of the original material remained. The principal factor in the receptive nature of this new research was related to the "profound and fundamental paradigm shifts" that displaced classical Newtonian physics along with their Cartesian philosophical counterpart. Replacing them, explained Christopher Kent Johannes, were "more encompassing and accurate views stemming from the quantum field, relativity, chaos, coherence, and holographic theories of the new physics and their expansive philosophical counterparts covered in holism, systems theory, ecological concepts and the informational paradigm."[45]

> The old universe of solid objects and deterministic laws of nature, with its linear time, arbitrary objectification and reductionism, was now dissolved into a universe of unbroken wholeness, wave-like patterns of interconnections and interweaving interacting probabilities, appearing as a dynamic web of inseparable energy patterns, in the dynamic matrix of a creative and infinitely intelligent eternal presentness. This scientific view of reality supports the homeopathic view of our dynamic energetic

> composition, nonlocal connections, the action of the non-material upon the material (and vice versa), our essential unitive kinship with the natural materia medica, and is consistent with the creatively teleological, self-maintaining, self-organizing, self-transcending nature attributed to the vital force that forms the essence behind our formal physical constitution and our life's dramatic scenarios.[46]

Finally, explained Johannes, the formation of a theoretical framework to explain the action of homeopathic medicinal agents was now within reach. Having recognized the misdirection of conventional models within the dominant biomedical paradigm, modern homeotherapeutists were now able to reconstitute Hahnemann's dynamic medicinal energies into a paradigm where the boundaries of science, metaphysics, spirituality, and theology blurred but where a small percentage of the world's scientists still remained much at home. It was here that the experiential, intuitive, and contemplative systems of East and West merged.[47]

Lurking in the shadows of homeopathy's high-energy medicine was the work of Amadeo Avogadro (1776-1856) on molecular weights. A contemporary of Hahnemann, he had published an article in the *Journal de physique* in 1811 demonstrating that a solute remained until approximately the 24X or 12C dilution. Beyond that, the chance that such a dilution contained even a single molecule of the solute was inconceivable.[48] Dilutions of this degree contained nothing but the liquid vehicle in which the substances were originally diluted and would act in no manner different from it. For homeopathy's critics, Avogadro's law stood as a formidable barrier to the claims of the high-potency advocates.[49]

For homeopaths, the prospect of dilutions beyond Avogadro's number had become a real possibility. Acknowledging that homeopathic solutions contained only water or alcohol, ultra-Avogadro medicines still had an ability to relieve symptoms of an illness in spite of the inability to identify the existence of substances in dilutions using standard laboratory techniques. According to Doctors G. P. Barnard and James H. Stephenson writing in 1978, Einstein's space-time continuum performed a crucial role in the biological sciences. The authors suggested that molecules called polymers that formed in a host's fluid were able to "reproduce themselves in the absence of the original substance which provoked their formation." Thus, an ultra-Avogadrian dilution (beyond 1×10^{-24}) would be chemically inert but nonetheless capable of transmitting its properties to a fixed and permanent substance. This required a shift to a three-dimensional view of the structure of ultra-Avogadrian dynamized serial dilutions. Borrowing from the work of English biochemists James D. Watson and Francis H. Crick on the structure of DNA, homeopaths argued that in a group of drugs of very similar chemical structure, even very small changes in the spatial arrangements of a molecule could alter toxicity. Homeopaths improvised with such terms as "chaos theory," "cohesive patterns," and "osotopic self-organization" to explain themselves, holding out for the ability to give a patient the structural content of a chemical without the actual chemical mass.[50]

This claim became a major bone of contention between homeopathy and regular medicine. For regular doctors, there was a point where further dilution interfered with the pharmacological action of the substance, decreasing its efficacy until what remained was nothing more than the vehicle of dilution. By contrast, homeopaths held that the dynamized substance altered the nature of the solution, dissolving chemical bonds and causing changes in its energy structure. Not surprisingly, this argument failed to appeal to the regular physician who countered that homeopathic medicines acted more from an intuitive "belief" than anything laboratory-based. To be sure, homeopaths had difficulty explaining themselves. In responding to the question how the energy of a remedy that was freed from its original physical vehicle acted as a cure, homeopaths were forced into a maze of verbal and metaphysical imprecisions:

> Dilution creates a regeneration system of dynamic rhythms, instead of the linear fading one would expect from the allopathic model. This establishes that energy specific to the remedy remains though no new molecules of the substance are present. Moreover, this energy is offered in pulses like breaths or heartbeats.[51]

Writing in the *JAIH* in 1978, Matthew Hubbard described the energy given off by a dilution as "a damped vibration, oscillating to the lower and lower levels as dilutions increase," but never stopping entirely. Considering that a drug's curative ability was a function of time and energy, the higher potencies would continue to work by virtue of their higher oscillations.[52]

> The energy is like a herald, signaling the presence of a substance, and upon ingestion, the organism, in its manifest levels, begins the series of actions necessary for removal of the intruder. But, of course, no physical intruder (or exceedingly little, in the lower potencies) has entered the system, and this series of actions (symptoms triggered by the remedy) instead work to clean the system of the already present ailment, whose similarity to the symptoms of the remedy determine the choice of curative agent. This unifies all of Hahnemann's postulates, showing that potentization can be proven essential to its two universally accepted predecessors, the law of similars and the law of the totality of the patient.[53]

In explaining how high-potency homeopathic remedies worked, Jacques Benveniste, a French immunologist, formulated a theory that when an original substance was diluted in pure water, the water retained a "memory" of its molecular structure despite its disappearance in the high dilutions. Michel Schiff in *The Memory of Water: Homeopathy and the Battle of Ideas in the New Science* (1995), detailed four years of experiments performed by Benveniste and his team of scientists. The team argued that water can remember its contact with biologically active substances. In other words, a drug's energy pattern was left in the water as a memory; it was not the substance that produced the effect, but the formative force or pattern of energy it carried. Benveniste's research was published in *Nature* in 1988 and resulted in an outpouring of scientific anger at editor John Maddox for allowing the report to be published. Along with complaints were accusations of fraud. Schiff's book described the subsequent investigations into the memory of water and of his conclusion that "the adamant refusal of scientists to enter into a serious discussion is an indication that there is something rotten in the kingdom of Academia."[54] Undeterred by the criticism, Benveniste opened a website to inform the public of his research and the field which he called "digital biology."[55]

CONTROLLED STUDIES

In explaining the present body of controlled studies on the effectiveness of homeopathic remedies, Doctors Daphna Slonim and Kerrin White of the Department of Psychiatry and the Behavioral Sciences at the University of California School of Medicine concluded in 1982 that homeopathy's clinical accounts generally "failed to follow current standards for case reporting" and therefore remained "outside" the mainstream of medical science. "To our knowledge," they wrote, "there exists no controlled, double-blind study comparing homeopathic treatment with any alternate treatment for a psychiatric disorder." While homeopathic literature abounded with case reports, few were written "convincingly enough to present to a skeptical audience." Most gave only anecdotal information and thus the results of homeopathic treatment were "lost" to the scientific community. There was also the issue of placebo effect in the review of evidence, particularly since the higher dilutions of homeopathic remedies contained no measurable amount of substance. This was an important issue because homeopathic remedies were often considered effective after a single application. Thus, the method of yielding a formal control group similar to conventional trials of mainstream medicine posed very idiosyncratic problems.[56]

In a review of fifty-nine homeopathic clinical trials published between 1945 and 1995, the Samueli Institute for Information Biology in Alexandria, Virginia, and the Department of Family Medicine at the Uniformed Services University of the Health Sciences in Bethesda, Maryland, showed that 29 percent used placebo controls and 51 percent used random assignment. The authors of the review concluded that clinical homeopathic research remained in its infancy "with most studies using poor sampling and measurement techniques, few subjects, single sites and no replication."[57]

Homeopaths attempted to counter the argument by asserting that their cures acted through the faith of the practitioner as transmitted to the patient. Essentially, each homeopathic drug had a unique quality or essence that was greater than its placebo effect. As David Taylor Reilly explained, when using the term placebo "we are really meaning successful self-healing, with all the complexity that implies." Homeopathy acted through the same pathways as self-healing and, as such, could enhance the placebo effect on patients. Although distinct, homeopathy and the placebo effect reinforced each other.[58]

For Jonathan Shore, MD, writing in 1990, the discussion raging around the placebo effect opened a whole new reordering of the relationship between the physician and the patient. Clearly, something dynamic existed between the intent of the physician, the psychophysiology of the patient, and the medicine. The issue was not simply whether the effect of homeopathic remedies was "just placebo," but whether homeopaths needed to have a better understanding of the criteria used to evaluate the efficacy of homeopathic remedies. Given the interaction between the medicinal substances which in their refined levels were "approaching that of mind itself," and the influence of mind or suggestion on the patient, the subtleties were such that "at any one moment it is almost impossible to say exactly to what degree the action of the substance administered is due to the activity of the substance or to the activity of mind, that is both the mind of the physician and that of the one who has come for assistance." How does one distinguish between placebo action and that of the active remedy? This reality placed in question the whole paradigm offered by regular medicine in its use of the placebo effect in drug trials.[59]

Thus homeopathic medicine became "not only a radically different system of therapeutics [but] also a radically different way of viewing the world," explained Karl Robinson, MD. Understanding it required a new paradigm, leaving behind most of nineteenth- and twentieth-century Cartesian thinking which emphasized logical thinking and a mechanistic interpretation of the universe. Although this older paradigm had brought many advances, it remained limited in its capacity.[60] As Bill Gray, MD, of California explained, "homeopathy operates on principles so diametrically opposed to allopathic medicine that we should not waste our limited efforts trying to convince irrelevant ivory-tower figures through double-blind studies, nor should we dance to the imagined tune of the increasingly irrelevant AMA."[61] This rather self-serving opinion, enunciated in 1992, was not too different from that spoken nearly a hundred years earlier. "You cannot measure homeopathy by the world's scientific standards because it is above them all," wrote the editor of the *Homeopathic Recorder* in 1899, "consequently one who attempts to judge the greater by the lesser will only land in confusion and skepticism."[62]

This view met with a trenchant response from the AMA. In its November 1998 issue on alternative medicine, the editors of *JAMA* wrote: "There is no alternative medicine. There is only scientific proven, evidence-based medicine supported by solid data or unproven medicine, for which evidence is lacking."[63] A similar statement came from an editorial in the *New England Journal of Medicine* (September 17, 1998) stating that "healing methods such as homeopathy and therapeutic touch are fervently promoted despite not only the lack of good clinical evidence of effectiveness, but the presence of a rationale that violates fundamental scientific laws."[64] Clearly, the so-called gold standard for research in modern medicine was the double-blind placebo clinical trial which, while criticized by many within the homeopathic community, held out the greatest potential for convincing skeptics of their alternative modalities.[65]

Unlike many of her colleagues, Jennifer Jacobs (b. 1950), a 1976 graduate of Wayne State University School of Medicine and professor of epidemiology at the University of Washington, believed that homeopathy lent itself to conventional randomized placebo-controlled trials. The reason for this, she argued, was that homeopathic medicines were given in lactose granules or pills which could be duplicated as placebo. "I believe it is possible to do highly rigorous scientific research in homeopathy and still retain the creative aspects of homeopathy," she wrote. This included individualization, the use of the placebo, and evaluating the whole person. Arguing against those in the homeopathic community who demanded an end to randomized clinical trials, Jacobs insisted that they were vital to the legitimacy of homeopathy and its standing in medicine. Anecdotal evidence had nowhere near the rigor necessary to justify homeopathy's integration into America's health care system.[66]

Jacobs hoped that the Center for Complementary and Alternative Medicine would consider funding more studies of homeopathy since, to date, only a handful had been supported.

> There is a good body of scientific evidence for homeopathy's effectiveness, especially in the area of clinical trials and meta-analyses, but apparently not enough to convince the skeptics. Priority should go to high methodological quality studies with adequate sample sizes to show significant effect sizes as well as

> to replication of previous studies by independent investigators. There are those who say that homeopathy will never be accepted until the mechanism of action is elucidated, which also would require a massive funding effort. Hopefully, this will come about through continued work within the NIH and other sources of governmental funding, as well as through private philanthropic organizations.[67]

In a chapter on homeopathy written by Jacobs and Richard Moskowitz in *Fundamentals of Complementary and Alternative Medicine* (1996), the two authors emphasized the Baconian nature of Hahnemann's scientific roots, the correlation between careful clinical symptomatology and the experimental pathogenesis of remedies, and the use of the single remedy and minimum dose, all being done under the overarching Law of Similia. American homeopathy had become a popular, safe, and effective alternative to the colossal third-party medical reimbursement system. The power, devotion, and vision of lay homeopaths had sustained homeopathy, leaving it to face three basic questions: Do highly dilute substances affect physical and biological systems? Can homeopathic medicines be proven to be effective clinically? What is the mechanism of action of homeopathic medicines?[68]

Recognizing that most scientists rejected homeopathic theory because of the nature of its extreme dilutions which extended far beyond the Avogadro limit of 10^{-24}, Jacobs and Moskowitz pointed to a hundred or more studies researching the effects of high dilutions in immunology, toxicology, and pharmacology. They recognized the conceptual difficulties present in many of the studies, some of which challenged the very tenets of biomedicine in their claims. They noted as well that there were fundamental impediments to doing clinical research in homeopathy due to its use of individualization of medicines, and that there was as yet "no scientific explanation for the mechanism of action of homeopathic medicines." The authors nevertheless hoped that developments in quantum physics and chaos theory might soon shed light on the electromagnetic interaction between the body and certain medicines even after the medicine was diluted to the point where it was no longer present in the menstrum. In looking at the subatomic world of new physics, they found themselves discovering particles of physical matter that were constantly appearing and disappearing. For them, contemporary biomedicine was conceptually dated using Newtonian and pre-Darwinian biology to explain its observations. By contrast, alternative and complementary medicine systems were recognizing new paradigms that accounted for wave functions, matter-energy duality, and a biology-ecology focus that engaged the inner resources of the patient in matters of health.[69]

Jacobs's efforts to turn homeopaths to double-blind clinical trials were not without opposition. In an extensive article in the *JAIH* in 2000, Richard Pitcairn explained to fellow homeopaths that modern allopathic medicine was without a coherent philosophy and that its two principal underpinnings—germ theory and the mechanical breakdown theory—were reductionist in nature, based on a philosophy of materialism, and out of touch with the physical, emotional, mental, and social context of the patient. Refusing to surrender to the philosophy of materialism, Pitcairn continued to adhere to a vitalistic life force or energy field that existed around living beings. Given that all physical objects were composed of fields of energy that vibrated through time and space, he considered it no stretch of the imagination to think that "living things may have a field of energy around them that is coincident with being 'alive.'" Pitcairn used this concept of life force to reject double-blind studies in scientific investigations, debunk treatment programs based on statistical analysis of patient groups or diagnostic categories, as well as all programs of palliation and suppression.[70] As long as regular medicine relied on palliative and reductionistic medicine as its primary means of treatment, and continued in economic league with pharmaceutical companies, insurance companies, and hospitals, homeopathy would remain steadfast in opposition.

Randall Neustaedter (b. 1940), speaking before the National Center for Homeopathy at its annual meeting in Chicago in 1987, thought it important for classical homeopaths to find a way to test the effectiveness of individualized treatment and not the allopathic test that analyzed a single specific medicine against a placebo. "If classical homeopathy advocates treating the totality of symptoms," he explained, "then it is clear that we cannot promote specifics. We must support studies that test the efficacy of homeopathic practice according to classical standards." He admitted that clinical double-blind controlled studies had their place, but he continued to push for "retrospective studies of cases from practice" as equally relevant. "After all," he explained, "the goal of clinical studies should be our own enlightenment, not vain attempts to convince the skeptic." By using journals, professional conferences, and computerized clinical reporting to provide information on clinical cases, he hoped that homeopaths would continue to build upon their materia medica as well as explain their prescribing styles to outsiders.[71]

By the mid-1990s, homeopathy's quest to build a rational medical science seemed lost in currents that were moving inexorably in the direction of a spiritual and metaphysical view of healing. Encouraged by a new group of lay leaders who provided novel answers to the inner harmony of the world of matter and the world of spirit, homeopaths moved further and further away from empirically tested systems of healing. In place of controlled clinical trials and more standardized medical practices, homeopaths opened themselves to a more mystical encounter between the individual and the cosmos, between the corporal body and the inner recesses of the mind. The uneasy truce between medicine and belief and between the academically trained physician and the laity had finally reached a crisis.

* * *

As explained by Andrew Weil, MD, this was the essence of the "irreconcilable philosophical difference" between homeopathy and conventional medicine. By refusing to accept that their medicines acted as placebos, homeopaths were insisting on "new physical and chemical laws" to explain the nature of their medicines' modus operandi. Obviously, this was a leap that reductionist science was unwilling to take without substantial justification grounded in sound empirical evidence.[72]

Chapter 5

Roads Taken and Not Taken

Given that the term "allopathy" had been originally intended as a derogatory description of mainstream medicine and connoted as a therapeutic regimen no longer practiced, editor Allan D. Sutherland (1897-1980) of the *JAIH* urged readers in the late 1950s to desist from using the word. Originally devised by Hahnemann in his bitterness, the term ignored medicine's empirical grounding as well as significant advances made during the middle and late nineteenth century.[1] Sutherland, a 1925 graduate of Hahnemann of Philadelphia and dean of the AIH Postgraduate School of Homeopathy from 1943 to 1979, was one of many at the AIH who hoped for a more collegial relationship in return for the acceptance of homeopathy as a therapeutic specialty within conventional medicine. Medicine was simply too big for any of its practitioners to cast aspersions at other practitioners, be they regular or homeopathic. Perhaps it was not much to hope that the day was not far distant when doctors of all schools would be happy to be known merely as physicians. The idea of homeopathy as a specialty, held since the founding of the Allentown Academy in 1836 and realized in European medical circles by the early twentieth century, had never been forgotten among America's more progressive homeopaths. Indeed, the hope that homeopathy would eventually be accepted by the American Medical Association as a legitimate choice of professional practice had long been the school's holy grail—a goal that routinely intersected its history from the early nineteenth to the end of the twentieth century. Ultimately, this long-held objective was dismantled by the leadership in the AMA as well as by lay leaders in the swelling ranks of Hahnemannians.

THE CULTIST THREAT

Henry W. Eisfelder, MD (d. 1975), a graduate of the New York Homeopathic College and member of the AIH board of trustees in 1955, liked the idea of homeopathy becoming a specialty but warned that it could easily become "a red flag before a bull." Remembering what had happened when homeopaths had permitted the AMA to rate their medical schools, he wondered if a similar trap might be lurking with this effort. More important to him was the pressing issue of new converts and the fact that, without change, "the practice of homeopathy in the United States . . . is doomed within another decade or two at the most." Fearing that laypersons were waiting to pick up where the professionals had left off, Eisfelder cautioned the AIH to prevent this from happening. The prospect of handing the reins of homeopathy over to the laity would most certainly bring harm, placing it among the more disreputable cults. Of imminent danger to the future of homeopathy was the threat of cultists seeking to enter the ranks of homeopathy by joining state homeopathic societies and then applying to take state board examinations. Most were chiropractors and naturopaths with degrees from schools not recognized by state licensing boards. Lamenting that some "benighted" members of the AIH might favor this backdoor approach to licensing, Eisfelder strongly opposed their admission. "If for no other reason than to protect us against such individuals," he urged the members of the AIH to fight "for the preservation of a homeopathy we may be proud to be associated with. . . . May we continue to merit the respect and admiration of all decent medical practitioners and not let our fair name be dragged in the mud."[2]

Others joined Eisfelder in warning of the efforts underway by irregular practitioners to gain control of homeopathy's nearly defunct state societies. "This is a situation which could be dangerous to the prestige of homeopathy and could reflect discredit of the AIH," wrote Allan D. Sutherland. If these associations were taken over by "spurious homeopaths," who had no valid MD degree, the AIH and its state associations could be stolen by "illegitimate children." To prevent this from happening, Sutherland urged state and county organizations to review their membership eligibility bylaws to ensure that no spurious doctors "crawl in through some crack." He thought it important to insist that applicants for membership be graduates of medical schools approved by the Council on Medical Education of the AMA and listed in the directory of the AMA.[3] In addition, Donald Gladish (1900-1967), president of the AIH in 1958, urged the elimination of defunct state boards to prevent their being used by those who were not homeopaths. These boards were unnecessary since there were no remaining medical schools teaching homeopathy whose graduates sought licensing. While the AIH lacked the statutory authority to force the closing of these boards, it went on record advising that it be done.[4]

During the 1950s, the AIH worked in unison with the AMA and the Federation of State Medical Boards to oppose the incursion of cultists and faith healers, many of whom were calling themselves homeopathic doctors and organizing homeopathic medical colleges and national homeopathic organizations. "They pose a particular threat to us," wrote Wyrth Post Baker, MD, "for they discredit us in the eyes of the medical profession and the public." It was time for homeopaths to divest themselves of their "paranoid delusions" of persecution by the AMA and join them to fight for the survival of private medical practice. "Unless immediate action is forthcoming," Baker warned, these newly organized colleges and associations would "revert by default to the cultist in another decade." Accordingly, he urged the establishment of a congress of homeopathic medical organizations no later than February 1958 to determine the standards for training and membership in their societies.[5]

As the AIH proceeded on a course that brought the organization into a closer working relationship with mainstream medicine, particularly in regard to licensing standards, Hahnemannians were equally aware of the need to maintain their separate identity. "We as homeopaths," wrote Henry W. Eisfelder, "must hew ever closer to the line of Hahnemannian principles if we are either to establish or to justify our right to a separate existence." This was especially important if homeopathy was to survive as a distinctive system. Allopathy with its reliance on the so-called miracle drugs—all of which contributed to the list of toxic symptoms—presented a position too divergent from the Law of Similia to permit any form of accommodation or synthesis. To the suggestion that homeopathy abandon its sectarianism and incorporate its knowledge into the broad field of medicine, Eisfelder responded quickly and to the point: "Don't let Homeopathy die!"[6]

Nevertheless, a premonition existed among AIH members that the medically licensed homeopath was a "vanishing American." The torch carried by homeopathy appeared to have passed to more receptive disciples in Great Britain, Mexico, Brazil, India, and Pakistan. In 1955, Paul S. Schantz, MD, who kept a card index of approximately 7,000 homeopathic physicians in the United States, noted that the last national directory had been published in 1941. Since then, natural attrition had reduced America's homeopaths to perilously low numbers.[7] In 1963, it was estimated that only about 1,590 medically trained physicians were practicing homeopathy in the United States.[8]

HOUR OF DECISION

In his president's message to the AIH in 1954, Arthur H. Grimmer, MD, informed members that the "hour of decision" was at hand. They had to choose whether "to perpetuate the only truly scientific system of medicine based on natural laws," or "abjectly surrender all the prerogatives and privileges" gained by their predecessors. Choosing the former, he urged their steps be "timed, synchronized and correlated to meet each and all of the numerous problems" they expected to confront.[9] Looking to the future, the AIH suggested six specific steps. These included: (1) the establishment of a Chronic Disease Board for the compilation of statistics on treatments; (2) the development of a homeopathic correspondence course available to licensed medical doctors; (3) annual progress reports from those doing research on homeopathic topics; (4) a memorial award for students doing original research in the field of homeopathic therapeutics; (5) development of a strong public relations program; and (6) joint officer meetings with lay organizations for better coordination and planning.[10]

With the ranks of both the AIH and the IHA depleted, there was renewed interest in merging the two organizations. Their separate existences may once have made sense due to fallacies that had crept into homeopathic practice, but the rationale for separate associations was no longer relevant.[11] In 1955, the president of the AIH formally proposed the amalgamation of the AIH, the Southern Homeopathic Medical Association, and the International Hahnemannian Association to form a new organization called the American Homeopathic Medical Association. The merger was advocated as a way of consolidating their individual strengths and thus enabling homeopathy to flex more weight in the world of medical politics.[12] With merger, the *Homeopathic Recorder,* which had been published for seventy-five years and had built a reputation for its devotion to pure Hahnemannian homeopathy, discontinued publication in 1959. In absorbing the *Homeopathic Recorder,* the *JAIH* began publishing more articles and reports emphasizing the symptomatic approach, together with more information on the teachings of Hahnemann and the other teachers of homeopathic philosophy and practice.[13]

Even with the disbanding of the IHA several obstacles remained unresolved. First and foremost was whether regular medicine would accept homeopathy as a legitimate specialty. Second, the vested interests and financial influence of the drug industry continued to weigh heavily on the side of regular medicine's drug-oriented culture. Third, there was the mental climate of the age, dubbed by some the "Aspirin Age," which symbolized all palliative drugs dispensed in a manner that homeopaths interpreted as degrading to the healing art. All three combined to create formidable obstacles to homeopathy's success.[14] In 1963, the AIH added to the list when it complained that the doctor-patient relationship was fast becoming passé. Group practice, clinics, nurses taking on physician's duties, and specialism had downgraded the general practitioner and led some to predict that trained laity would soon replace the general practitioner.[15]

By the mid-1960s, most American homeopaths were in agreement that their earlier endeavor to build and operate colleges at a cost of many millions of dollars had ended in catastrophe. Convinced that homeopathic therapeutics would be better working *within* the ranks of medicine and not as a separate school, most concluded to never again build another college. "The education of the medical student is no business of ours," wrote William W. Young, MD (1900-1974), of Ohio, and this error must never be repeated. All that the colleges produced were a "few graduates who knew some materia medica and who, after graduation, either became experts or forgot what they learned." Otherwise, they produced little in the way of research data, scholarly treatises, or academic accomplishments. Indeed, argued Young, the most skilled members of homeopathy had almost always come from regular colleges.[16]

Young, a graduate of Hahnemann of Philadelphia in 1928, noted that over the previous seventy years the medical curriculum had undergone enormous change. Indeed, the breadth and depth of what medical students were required to learn had increased exponentially. During that time, numerous specialties had found their place while others had come and gone. During that same period, however, homeopathic curriculum had stayed much the same. What was taught decades earlier was the same today, and for Young, this was unacceptable. Not only was the homeopathic curriculum "archaic" and "antediluvian," it "has been and still is moribund, static inert." Its foundational work remained dependent upon the writings of a man who lived and wrote at the time of George Washington.[17] In addition, there were few if any experiments demonstrating the objective proof of the tenets of homeopathy and no authoritative texts. Instead, there was a "Babel of tongues, a chaos of conflicting opinions, a conflict of personal animosities." Faced with these impediments, Young urged his fellow homeopaths to adapt. Socialized medicine, medicare, group practice, and the free clinic were the obvious signs of the time and homeopaths had either to accept these new realities or leave the profession. Nevertheless, if homeopathy was to exist as a medical specialty, it was necessary "to adopt an aggressive policy of education." This required an extensive review of the medical literature, much of which had been neglected for more than a century. Beyond this, it was necessary for certain individuals or groups to take on the responsibility for educating those interested in advancing the cause of homeopathy.[18]

Instead of seeking to establish the medical college model, Young followed in the steps of his predecessors by urging that homeopathy be accepted as part of the curriculum in mainstream medical colleges. This could be done through the creation of chairs or lectureships which allowed for the recognition of homeopathy as a medical philosophy and a pharmaco-therapeutic method. Young noted that in 1965, the president of the AMA had been a guest speaker at the national convention of the AIH. Although he had never expected to witness such a visit during his lifetime, its significance was not lost. "I interpret it as signifying an interest in, a sympathy toward and a curiosity about that for which we stand and that it also signifies an opportunity," Young remarked. It represented not an endorsement of homeopathic methods or philosophy but as a "willingness to listen to what we have to say."[19]

Hoping that his colleagues would decide that lectureships were the appropriate "instrument of choice," Young urged that a process be undertaken to find suitable candidates whose specialties were in medicine, pharmaco-therapeutics, biology, organic, colloidal or physical chemistry, neurology, or basic medical research. A committee of the AIH would have the responsibility to identify, hire, and report the activities of such lectureships annually. Out of these efforts he hoped would emerge an up-to-date scientific and well-documented literature bearing directly on homeopathy. To accomplish this task, he urged the merging of the various trusts and endowments that had been used to support past homeopathic colleges. These funds, once located and combined with newer endowments, could be used to support the proposed lectureships.[20]

MEMBERS ONLY

In remarks before the AIH in 1979, Frederic Schmidt, MD, of California questioned whether the association should adhere to the old bylaws that limited membership to medical doctors, osteopathic physicians and dentists, or whether it should allow licensed naturopaths, chiropractors, and PhDs in related health disciplines to become members. Equally important, should the AIH support the re-establishment of new medical colleges? Or, should homeopathic courses such as those offered by George Vithoulkas represent the "promised land" for homeopathy's future? Transition to a higher level of knowledge could not occur if well-trained homeopaths were unavailable. By the same token, increasing the numbers of nonmedically degreed homeopaths could force new restrictions on homeopathy, including its re-classification as a nonmedical therapy. If the solution was to increase the numbers of "pseudo-doctors [who] latched onto homeopathy and feel quite competent after reading a few books," then, Schmidt feared, great harm would come to the profession.[21]

Schmidt ended his presidential duties in 1980 with a letter to AIH members asking for an explanation why the association's memberships were decreasing at a time when interest in homeopathy was "bursting out of its seams all across the country?" He pointed out that homeopathic colleges were being born "either for real or on paper" in states from Connecticut to Florida, New Mexico, and California; that lectures and seminars on homeopathy were being sponsored by lay groups, naturopaths, and chiropractors; and that holistic associations and ad hoc homeopathic societies were organizing and advertising memberships open to all. Schmidt expressed alarm at these unauthorized activities. "Should people with limited backgrounds of medical sciences blithely treat long-standing or chronic illnesses, the seriousness of which they may not be aware, and the consequences of which they cannot foresee, or take care of when they occur?" he asked rhetorically. Alternatively, "Should we be contented to be a small rugged group of medically trained physicians, organized in the medical tradition of the AIH, or should we follow the trend of the times, and move away from what we learned? Shall we abdicate clinical medicine, and the knowledge of clinical Homeopathy?" Schmidt, who had been in practice for more than thirty years, refused to countenance these "new prophets" who seemingly "leased" homeopathy as the vehicle for spreading their particular form of "energy medicine." He pointed out that this problem had first risen with the Liga Medicorum Homeopathica Internationalis (LIGA) which included a number of "new medicine" doctors and laypersons whose enthusiasm seemed unequaled. However, Schmidt refused to support a change in AIH membership even if it meant extinction. He feared that these new "young doctors" would, if accepted into the ranks, seek leadership of the organization. If this happened, homeopathy would become "a thing of the past" and the word "medical" would forever be omitted from its mission. In the end, he warned, these "short-cut energy practitioners" would destroy classical homeopathy. "We must survive and preserve what we inherited from our great homeopathic teachers," he concluded, "in order to hand over an intact organization to those who come after us."[22]

Jack Cooper, MD (1917-1987), who succeeded Schmidt as president of the AIH in 1980, signaled a change in direction when he suggested that the association should consider amending its rules of admission. While Schmidt had emphasized "togetherness," Cooper emphasized "growth." Like others in the AIH, Cooper desired that homeopathy become a specialty in the practice of medicine and that pure homeopathy be kept alive for posterity; but he also openly advocated a more inclusive membership.[23] Cooper's position reflected the views of a growing sector within the broader homeopathic community willing to acknowledge that naturopaths, acupuncturists, masseurs, nutritionists, and chiropractors had been on the front lines and responsible for keeping homeopathy alive as a healing art. Had Hahnemann intended for homeopathy to be practiced only by medical doctors, reasoned Hela Michot-Dietrich, PhD, of New York, he would have written his books in Latin rather than in German. Besides, one of Hahnemann's principal disciples had been Clemens Maria Franz von Boenninghausen (1785-1864) who had his doctorate in civil and criminal law, not medicine. Having felt betrayed by those who insisted that healing should reside in the exclusive domain of licensed physicians, Michot-Dietrich put her faith in the lay practitioners of homeopathy.

> What is it that makes presumably-educated people believe that they have cornered the truth and that no one not carrying the official seal of good quality should have access to this same truth? The right to the pursuit of happiness guaranteed under the Constitution of the United States allows the public to seek good health, so important an ingredient to happiness in this world, wherever and from whomever they can get it. If the information on making atomic weapons is readily accessible to all who know where to find it, why should not that on healing one's fellow creatures be available to all?[24]

Among the many newcomers who urged changes in the membership requirements for the AIH was Julian Winston, associate professor of Design and Theory at the Philadelphia College of Art, who explained that the demise of the homeopathic medical schools in the United States "came about because *credentials* were looked at in place of *knowledge*." In other words, the abilities of applicants had been supplanted by the rating of the school. Believing that more than half of the "respected" homeopaths practicing in the United States in the 1980s fell outside the above rankings, Winston urged the AIH to reconsider its admission policies and practices.[25]

The uneasy truce over AIH membership broke in 1988 when Jacquelyn Wilson, the association's new president, recommended a rule change allowing admission of acupuncturists, naturopaths, chiropractors, nurse-practitioners, and nurses who practiced homeopathy. The recommendation elicited an immediate response from Franklin

McCoy, MD, of Greenwich, Connecticut, who reported that when he first joined the Connecticut Homeopathic Medical Society there were only six other members. They included three practicing MDs, two physicians who practiced no homeopathy "but enjoyed discussing football," and a psychiatrist who was a "diploma-mill graduate, not a licensed physician," and for whom the bylaws had been changed to accommodate his membership. Soon after joining the society, the psychiatrist began lobbying for licensure as a homeopathic physician. This, McCoy warned, was clear evidence of what would soon engulf the field of homeopathy if the rule was allowed to change.[26] Similarly, Domenick John Masiello, DO, of New York, complained that a group of local anthroposophical physicians had joined a small group of self-styled "complementary" physicians to restore the dormant Homeopathic Medical Society of the State of New York.* Their purpose was to afford legal protection for their peculiar therapeutic practices by calling themselves homeopathic. This, Masiello argued, was contrary to the basic tenets of homeopathy and he hoped the AIH would take a stand against the society's recognition.[27]

Again in 1991, Edward Chapman, MD, the incoming president of the AIH, asked for an open discussion on the purpose of the organization and its rules on membership. The AIH, he explained, represented MDs, osteopaths, and dentists and, as such, was primarily a "trade organization" designed to protect the practice of homeopathy. Over the years, the AIH had formed coalitions with other organizations to accomplish a meaningful legislative agenda. During that same period, the homeopathic community had changed significantly, with patients prescribing for themselves, their families, and even others outside the immediate family. "Homeopathy generates a patient-centered system, where patients become empowered to heal themselves," explained Chapman. While this self-help system threatened traditional boundaries of professional training, he nonetheless found it refreshing in its openness and urged the AIH to look at its "standards of practice" with the commitment to expanding AIH's membership, thereby giving the organization the critical mass needed to accomplish its work.[28]

---

*Founded by Rudolf Stiner (1861-1925) and further enhanced by Ita Wegman (1876-1943), this school of medicine aims to treat the body as well as the mind, spirit, and soul. The four parts cooperate within the nerve-sense, rhythmic, and metabolic systems.

Chapman's decision to open discussion on membership was followed by a challenge over the AIH requirement that, to be eligible for membership, physicians be in an active homeopathic practice. Recognizing that their medicine had grown in both lay and professional practices, it was important, Guy Hoagland, MD, argued, to ask how homeotherapeutics was perceived in its historical relationship with old school medicine. As defined at the state and federal levels, homeotherapeutics was "the application of homeopathic drugs in the clinical practice of medicine." This definition left out a number of critical elements (i.e., single dose, dynamization) but gave broad applicability for both the trained physician and the untrained prescriber. Hoagland viewed homeotherapeutics as a pyramid with generalists providing a broad base of primary or grass-roots support. "The primary care practitioners may know little of the philosophies of Hahnemann or Kent," he explained, "but they can know Arnica for first-aid cases, Ignatia for appropriate cases of acute grief reactions, and combination medicines for other minor, self-limited conditions." Held in poor regard by specialists, they were nonetheless a useful source of referral that supported a "second tier" of practitioners who specialized in homeotherapeutics. Above them was a "third tier" of practitioners considered for their training, expertise, and insight into specialty areas. Hoagland recognized the interdependence of the three levels in the pyramid and that, to be effective, each of the levels would require tolerance and mutual respect. "Today there are many philosophies and empiric determinations of practice that are included in the specialty of homeotherapeutics," he explained. "When held in mutual respect, they provide the dynamic tension of professional challenge that is necessary for growth and excellence."[29]

Because the modern practice of homeopathy in the United States lay in the hands of so many untrained practitioners outside the mainstream of regular medical practice, questions continued to be raised within and outside the AIH as to whether homeopathy was truly a medicine, or whether it had become more of a religion. For Hoagland, modern homeopathy had "transcended" medical training and was fast becoming a religion rather than a scientifically based therapeutical system of medicine. "The focus on healing as a primarily personal and experiential phenomenon in treatment with homeopathic medicine lacks a fundamental scientific basis," he admitted, "and promotes homeopathy as a religious experience, not as a sound medical practice."[30] As explained by Hoagland, lay homeopathy focused on the materia medica, repertory, and case analysis without instruction on patient evaluation relative to diagnosis, prognosis, and the parameters of management. "It is wrongly assumed," he reasoned, "that these issues are either irrelevant or magically conferred on the student in the study of the homeopathic prescription for illness." For Hoagland, there was a clear distinction between individualization in the application of a scientific treatment method and the personal experience of healing. In the latter situation, the application of the healing art "has no basis in scientific principle." This approach or mindset presupposed that homeopathic education was "transcendent" over all other medical training. Such a mindset "weakens the promotion and development of homeotherapeutics as a reproducible, scientific, and legitimate medical treatment method." With no more substance than belief, lay homeopaths were pursuing a path that defied "common sense" and "good clinical judgment."[31]

In Hoagland's estimation, homeopathy's broad community of practitioners had to decide if they wanted to continue promoting homeopathy as a scientifically based medical practice, or "openly define homeopathy as a religion beyond science."

> If the latter, homeopathy should clearly be presented as a religious cult and guidelines should be developed for interacting with the secular and scientific world. If homeopathy is defined as a method of homeotherapeutics, consisting of pharmaceutical products, a body of demonstrable, reproducible facts, and principles that are not dependent on a particular philosophical orientation a priori, it can be a medical specialty that will grow with the expanding limits of scientific investigation and clinical expertise. When presented as a science, it is founded in scientific method with an openness to be tested in multiple world views, philosophies and theories.[32]

As the individual most responsible for initiating the discussion, Chapman lamented Hoagland's characterization of homeopathy as a field divided by "we and they" and "religion and science." This way of thinking, he cautioned, "has never helped and has only served to divide the homeopathic community." While Chapman sought to build a greater consensus among nonmedical caregivers, he was troubled that the "MD" degree carried such a negative connotation among these advocates, and particularly against those doctors who had entered homeopathy by way of allopathic medicine. The homeopathic movement was too small, he felt, to be divided. There must be mutual respect and acceptance among homeopathy's many elements. "For us," Chapman argued, "the development of allopathic competency has not been an end, but a foundation."[33]

Chapman's concern for greater civility was due, in part, to Randall Neustaedter's fear of what he perceived as a trend within the AIH to "court the allopath." Neustaedter, one of the originators of the Bay Area Homeopathic Study Group in 1972, had cautioned the homeopathic community on the dangers of those among them who "sought approval from the allopaths" of their ideas. It was important to recognize that "the fate of homeopathy does not rest with MDs anymore," he proclaimed. Even though the old guard of homeopathic MDs had insisted on keeping homeopathy elitist and closed to newer ideas, the best work of modern homeopathy on the materia medica had come from George Vithoulkas, Paul Herscu (b. 1959), Catherine Coulter (b. 1934), and Ananda Zaren; and on the repertory from David K. Warkentin (b. 1951), and Forrest Murphy. These works, he explained, these were not the products of MDs but of laypersons. The hope of homeopathy someday becoming a medical specialty and given the "keys to the allopathic kingdom," was no longer a worthy objective, Neustaedter believed. This long-held hope of the "holy grail" among old guard homeopaths was neither realistic nor valid. Given the fact that regular medicine never absorbed, integrated, or accepted homeopathy, and had only wanted to "conquer and destroy it," the AIH had been wrong in its quest to seek allopathic approval. Allopaths, Neustaedter concluded, "can no more recognize the existence and legitimacy of homeopathy than medieval astronomers could admit that the earth was not the center of the universe."[34]

Not surprisingly, there was considerable disagreement over Neustaedter's remarks. That the fate of homeopathy no longer rested with MDs and that allopathy was undeserving of respect were bellicose claims deemed unwarranted by Karl Robinson, MD (b. 1938), editor of the *JAIH* from 1984 to 1990. In defense of allopathy, he remarked.

> All of us, at one point or another, are glad to have allopathy around. When someone needs surgery, thank God surgeons and operating rooms exist. When someone has advanced asthma and the homeopath is not finding the correct remedy, thank God for inhalers and adrenaline. When the homeopath, for lack of skill or luck, cannot find the correct remedy in an advancing pneumonia, thank God for antibiotics. . . . My gripe with allopathy is that it has preempted all other non-emergency areas of medicine, particularly chronic illness when one or another of the complementary medical specialties would be far more effective. I would like to see the alternative/complementary fields of medicine seeing 60 to 70 percent of patients instead of 5 to 10 percent as we do now. That is the problem. The ratio is wrong.[35]

Even in the mid-1990s, with approximately 2,000 physicians practicing homeopathy in the United States and with their belief system growing, the AIH could claim little more than one hundred members. Fearing charges of elitism from non-MD colleagues, and noticing the popularity of homeopathic remedies used by naturopaths, chiropractors, nurse-practitioners, physician-assistants, nurses, acupuncturists, psychotherapists, midwives, lay educators, and counselors, the AIH found itself facing pragmatic questions about its future. With the National Center for Homeopathy representing both professionals and laypersons, and the Homeopathic Community Council working to establish uniform standards of conduct, practice, and accreditation for nonmedically qualified caregivers, the question came down to whether the continued existence of the AIH was really necessary. For Richard Moskowitz, MD, the answer was clear. To survive, the AIH had an obligation to support nonhomeopathic colleagues as equals within the profession. Despite issues dealing with certification and licensure, and essential disagreements over methodology (highs vs. lows; unicists vs. pluralists; and differences among charismatic teachers, radioesthetists, dowsers, and electro-diagnosticians), he felt it possible for all to come together on "how we relate to our patients" and on standards of accountability. No doubt homeopathy would be far different in years to come. Recognizing the importance and perils of both the known and the unknown, homeopaths had to build bridges among themselves.[36]

The growing popularity of alternative health and self-care movements coincided with the spiraling cost of regular medicine in the 1990s. Their new visibility also exposed a number of issues that homeopaths found hard to ignore. This included the crass advertising of homeopathic remedies for baldness, impotence, and similar disorders; the use of "outlandish" slogans; the encouragement of illegal or unlicensed devices; and the lack of informed consent and basic disregard for standards of care. All of this was made even more complicated because there was no separate homeopathic profession recognized by law "and characterized by uniform standards of education and training," including a code of ethics. Instead, homeopathy was being practiced by all types of caregivers, each with their respective licensing or certifying boards, educators, and advocates. Under these circumstances, it was difficult to imagine an ethics code "sufficiently uniform and rigorous to enforce meaningful discipline, yet flexible enough to accommodate such a wide range of needs and experience." Homeopaths needed a code to help bring these groups together "to constitute a profession that does not yet exist." For Moskowitz, the creation of a code would enable homeopaths to suspend their differences in methods and practices and "affirm what we all have in common, namely, a patient-centered philosophy of healing and the healing relationship that the medical profession is in stark need of at the moment."[37]

At issue was if and in what manner the AIH could connect its many and diverse healing communities. Complicating this task was the prevalent belief among nonprofessional caregivers that the MD degree had been an impediment to the full understanding of homeopathy. Finding a middle ground between the medically educated homeopath and the nonmedically qualified healer was a challenge that went to the very heart of AIH's future. At the time, no middle ground existed. The American Board of Homeotherapeutics (ABHT) certified the qualifications of MDs and DOs, and the Homeopathic Academy of Naturopathic Physicians (HANP) certified NDs who practiced homeopathy. The ABHT was incorporated in 1960 and patterned after the guidelines established by the Advisory Board for Medical Specialties of the AMA. Its examination replicated that of the Faculty of Homeopathy in London, consisting of a three-part process that included the submission of ten treated chronic cases with follow-up; a written examination; and an oral examination. Maintaining the Diplomate status also required continuing education credits as well as articles submitted for publication in the *JAIH*.[38]

Chapman took note of the Primary Care Physician Education Project, cosponsored by the AIH and the Academic Faculty of Glasgow Homeopathic Hospital, which introduced a course on the basic concepts of homeopathy to serve as a means of credentialing. This postgraduate course had run successfully in Scotland for twelve years, requiring 40 classroom and 80 home study hours, and ending with an examination which served as the basis for a Primary Care Certificate. Chapman urged its implementation in the United States, explaining that it could serve as a base level credentialing for insurance companies, managed care organizations, and hospitals. If carried out, it would permit homeopathy to migrate into the medical mainstream. A pilot program was initiated in March 1996 in San Francisco to test whether the concept could be used in the United States as successfully as it had been used in the United Kingdom.[39]

For nonmedically qualified practitioners, the Council for Homeopathic Certification (CHC) offered an examination process. As for certifying institutions, the Council on Homeopathic Education (CHE) was the body to which all educational institutions could apply for accreditation. No matter whether the program was designed for MDs, DDSs, NDs, RNs, chiropractors, OMDs, physician assistants, or certified acupuncturists, the council was the central agency for all licensed disciplines requiring continuing education. By 1990, only three had applied for accreditation: the National College of Naturopathic Medicine, the International Foundation for Homeopathy, and the National Center for Instruction of the National Center for Homeopathy.

As homeopathy gained in popularity in the 1990s, Chapman grew increasingly concerned with the challenges ahead. Among them were the need for more scientific substantiation of homeopathic remedies; more information on homeopathy's cost-effectiveness; an examination of labeling requirements for homeopathic medicines; and the need for certification and licensing. He argued persuasively that hospitals, managed care organizations, and insurers were legitimately demanding some level of credentialing to justify proper assessment and payment of services. While the ABHT credentialed MD and DO physicians with the title of Diplomate of Homeotherapeutics, similar credentialing was needed elsewhere among providers of homeopathic services. Many were eligible for this certification, but he noted that only sixty practitioners were certified with the Diplomates of the American Board of Homeotherapeutics and the same number for the Diplomates of the Homeopathic Association of Naturopathic Physicians. About hundred were certified by the CHC, and about twenty Diplomates were certified by the North American Society of Homeopaths. The gap between what was possible and what existed suggested two explanations: either homeopaths were not "joiners" or they failed to see the value in certification.[40]

HOMEOPATHIC PHARMACOPOEIA

From 1888 through the eighth edition (1979) of the *Homeopathic Pharmacopoeia of the United States,* the publication resided in the hands of the AIH. The 1938 Food Drug and Cosmetic Act recognized the FDA's right to regulate homeopathy. The author of this act, Royal B. Copeland, was a homeopathic physician who wished to see homeopathy perpetuated. For Copeland, the perpetuation of homeopathy required the FDA to first regulate it; and by choosing to regulate it, the FDA would then be forced to recognize it.[41]

Because the *Homeopathic Pharmacopoeia of the United States* was recognized in law as having equal status with the *United States Pharmacopoeia* and because most states required either the MD or DO degree for the practice of medicine, the prescriptions derived from the homeopathic pharmacopoeia were reserved only for licensed physicians. If, however, laypersons chose to practice medicine, the AIH warned that homeopathy would have to be reclassified as "non-medical therapy." This would require homeopathy to change its status from a drug-based therapeutic system to something akin to physiotherapy, nutrition, or other adjuncts to medicine. "The legal sanction of lay homeopathic practice on the grounds that 'holistic health-care' is not medicine and Homeopathy is a part of this holistic healthcare, inevitably means that Homeopathy is no longer a proper medical drug therapy," explained the editor of the *JAIH.* Clearly, homeopathy was in a state of "disorder," "confusion," and "rapid change."[42]

The market resurgence in the 1970s paved the way for industry growth in the 1980s and opened homeopathy to many new aggressive drug companies in addition to old-line houses. With this new market, however, came the introduction of many semi-homeopathic remedies. In order to avoid being sued for noninclusion of these remedies, many of which the AIH wanted no part, the AIH permitted the separate incorporation of the Homeopathic Pharmacopoeia Convention of the United States to publish the ninth edition in 1982.[43]

In 1986, the homeopathic industry was approached by the FDA with a request for another regulatory proposal. This triggered the creation by the American Association of Homeopathic Pharmacists of the Joint Action Committee for negotiating with the FDA. Some of the issues included the following: What makes a product homeopathic? What distinguishes an official from an unofficial or over-the-counter (OTC) homeopathic product? Why were homeopathic labels in Latin? Why were not homeopathic single remedies labeled with complete indications? Are there homeopathic medicines which must be distributed by prescription only? These questions were the result of the multitude of OTC remedies sold through the mail or in retail outlets. The Joint Action Committee attempted to play down the distinctions between official and unofficial products. In doing so, it attempted to find a middle ground by arguing that unofficial drugs were negligible. If accepted by the FDA, companies would be able to market homeopathic products without fear of regulatory changes.[44]

Although the AIH saw a favorable climate on the horizon, much of this was due to the downsizing of the FDA and the fact that its personnel were reluctant to take on further regulation. However, the AIH saw problems with the National Council Against Health Fraud (NCAHF), formed in 1984, which had asked the FDA to require "that all OTC homeopathic drugs meet the same standards of safety and effectiveness as non-homeopathic OTC drugs." While the petition represented a major challenge to homeopathy in that these products were the mainstay of numerous homeopathic pharmacies, President Sandra M. Chase, MD, of the AIH saw the petition as bringing ultimate regulation to the products being marketed. Some of these unregulated products were being manufactured "by who knows whom" and under labels that promised miracle cures. Many, too, contained multiple ingredients and were highly toxic. Besides, classically oriented homeopaths were not the only ones alarmed at the explosion of these products. Traditional herbalists were concerned that the medicines were being mass produced and marketed by whoever had the imagination and capital to do so. "We know that we are dealing with powerful and effective medicines, which while natural are not candy or placebos," commented Chase. "Just as the overuse of antibiotics endangers their effectiveness, the same may be true for our products."[45]

Edward Chapman continued to raise concerns with the public face of homeopathy, fearing that its lack of standards would lead to problems of safety and proper labeling in homeopathic remedies; greater scrutiny on efficacy and mechanism of action; and increased demands from regulatory agencies, hospitals, and managed care entities for assurances of competence. Until the homeopathic community addressed these issues, conventional medicine would continue to fight the claims of alternative medicine. "My goal," Chapman explained, is "to see homeopathy become part of the primary medical care of all Americans."[46]

Fearing the heightening wrath of the National Council Against Health Fraud which was demanding closer scrutiny of homeopathy by the FDA, Chapman continued to speak out for greater accountability. At the heart of the council's criticism was that homeopathic products were being sold on the OTC market with labels suggesting efficacious treatment for many different complaints. Nevertheless, homeopathic products were not required to demonstrate their clinical efficacy on the assumption that, having been used for more than two hundred years, "the public should be free to choose as long as there is no risk." Further complicating the issue was the FDA's decision to waive its phase one and two studies of homeopathic medicines and permit researchers to go directly to a phase three, efficacy trial. Because homeopathy challenged the basic tenants of biomedical medicine, Chapman believed it was no longer wise for homeopaths to ignore criticism. He urged homeopaths to support the FDA in developing a better labeling of homeopathic products; urged the designing and conducting of basic homeopathic science experiments "to define and measure the activity of homeopathic medicine in biological systems"; and supported the use of clinical trials "to prove the general validity of classical homeopathy as a method of treating a number of clinical situations." Overall, he argued, it was important to lay aside fears and self-interest and to embark on a constructive dialogue with the FDA "that rises above idolatry and uses what is best in science and the regulatory system to bring the public a safe and effective medicine."[47]

QUESTIONABLE LEGITIMACY

Unfortunately, the gap between homeopathy's popularity and its unlicensed entrepreneurial healers created serious problems of legitimacy at the very moment when a combination of social and economic factors was encouraging homeopathy's growth and popularity as a valued commodity. This new attention had a double edge to it. Homeopaths seemed willing to bathe in the light of their new recognition, but that same popularity focused attention on the lack of validation for many of the clinical claims made by both caregivers and pharmaceutical manufacturers—all the more reason to implement some form of certification, accreditation, and licensure. The OTC status of homeopathic medicines allowed them to be prescribed by all—from medical and osteopathic physicians, podiatrists, dentists, chiropractors, acupuncturists, naturopaths, oriental medical doctors, nurse-practitioners, physician-assistants, and pharmacists, to dieticians, cosmetologists, and laypersons. Indeed, lay practitioners such as George Vithoulkas, Catherine Coulter, Lou Klein, Henne gutten Mast, and Jeremy Sherr, to mention only a few, felt confident enough to prescribe "professionally." This latitude created a legitimate level of uncertainty in the status of the professional homeopath in the United States. How, Edward Chapman asked, does one determine if a professional homeopath is practicing in the appropriate manner? The time was fast approaching when issues would arise involving professional identity, education, and regulation. When that happened, the issues would "transcend the jurisdiction of any person or organization within the homeopathic community." In Minnesota, for example, professional homeopathy was treated outside the scope of the state's medical practices act. This meant that the state would not interfere with these non-medically licensed practitioners so long as they did not represent themselves as physicians or attempt to diagnose and treat disease. As of 2000, only Arizona, Connecticut, Delaware, Nevada, and New Hampshire had extended to homeopaths some degree of regulation.[48]

For Chapman, it was essential for America's practicing homeopaths to seek legitimacy through some form of credentialing, accreditation, or licensure. Unless this was done, homeopathy's popularity would be unsustainable. How this was handled would ultimately affect the AIH and its debate over membership. The AIH's willingness to change its eligibility rules would ultimately depend upon the willingness of homeopathy's caregivers to commit themselves to a process that molded the profession into a cadre of well-trained, licensed practitioners with established standards of certification.[49] In Chapman's parting words as president of the AIH, he warned that governments around the world were asking homeopathy "to get its act together, not only around pharmacy issues, but also setting criteria for education and certification."[50]

In October 1998, the AIH board of trustees approved the addition of a new class of "associated members" for licensed advanced practice nurses and licensed physician's assistants.[51] However, having made this concession, the AIH found itself hard pressed to close the gates. As a result, homeopaths of all stripes demanded entry. When Jennifer Jacobs, MD, president of the AIH in 2001, remarked that homeopathy was "a medical practice that requires a balance between mind and heart, art and science, the practical, focused left brain mode of thinking with the more intuitive, subjective feelings attributed to right brain consciousness," she gave official blessing to AIH's newest transients.[52]

Jacobs claimed significant accomplishments under her leadership of the AIH. Not only was the *JAIH* issued in a whole new format, including a new name (*American Journal of Homeopathic Medicine*), but the AIH grew in membership; increased its offerings of seminars, conferences, and primary care courses for medical professionals; instituted a speaker's bureau for lay and professional groups; developed new promotional materials; and established a presence with governmental and regulatory agencies, including the White House Commission on Complementary and Alternative Medicine (CAM) and the NIH's Office of Alternative Medicine (OAM).[53] In reflecting on the twenty-five years since she had become interested in homeopathy, Jacobs recalled the excitement in the 1970s and early 1980s when the San Francisco Bay Area study groups were in full swing. "Since that time," she observed, "homeopathy has grown, but not flourished." Although it was hard to speculate on the reasons, she noted that some had moved in the direction of clinical research while others explored new methods of prescribing or carrying out provings. Nevertheless, while other CAM modalities had grown in popularity, homeopathy seemed "in danger of falling off the radar screen." Exemplary of this, the NIH successor to OAM, the National Center for Complementary and Alternative Medicine, chose to fund very few studies on homeopathy. The reason for this stemmed from homeopathic efforts to justify the irrelevance of randomized and placebo-controlled research trials as applicable to classical homeopathy.[54]

Rather than accept infighting as the cause of homeopathy's problems, Jacobs countered that "homeopathy is so revolutionary in its concept, so 'outside the box' of the current medical paradigm," that it could not fit into the commercial and popular notion of "complementary," "alternative," or "integrative" medicine. The irony, she explained, was that in an era of spiraling costs in mainstream medicine, homeopathy was not something that could be used—like acupuncture—as an adjunct to conventional medicine. It could not be mass marketed. Instead, it stood alone as a "cohesive philosophy of health and disease."[55] In her comments before the White House Commission on Complementary and Alternative Medicine, Jacobs claimed there was sufficient research to justify the use of homeopathy in numerous medical conditions. While its modus operandi remained a question mark, she suggested that it "most likely [worked] on a subatomic or subtle energy level that [had] not yet been elucidated."[56]

COLLEGE TRAINING

In 1985, the National College of Naturopathic Medicine in Portland, Oregon, and the John Bastyr College of Naturopathic Medicine in Seattle, Washington, began offering homeopathy as part of their curriculum along with botanical medicine, Oriental medicine, hydrotherapy, clinical nutrition, spinal manipulation, counseling, and exercise therapy. Training required the study of homeopathy for one full year, or, alternatively, seven semesters over the course of the entire program.[57] Eventually, all naturopathic medical schools supported a department or program in classical Hahnemannian philosophy. Being a naturopathic doctor, however, was no guarantee of competence in homeopathy. Those wishing to be competent had to spend additional time learning homeopathic philosophy as well as clinical therapeutics. A substantial number of naturopathic doctors enrolled in postgraduate homeopathic seminars. The Homeopathic Academy of Naturopathic Physicians (HANP), with its journal *Simillimum,* was a specialty society of naturopaths that worked to strengthen the practice of homeopathy within the profession.[58]

In 1992, there were approximately 1,000 licensed naturopathic physicians practicing in the United States.[59] Together, they counted as a significant sector of the homeopathic community with many having specialized in homeopathic practice. Representing this group was the American Association of Naturopathic Physicians (AANP) which not only lobbied for protective legislation, but fought to ensure that their educational standards were met. Both Bastyr and National College were accredited by the Council on Naturopathic Medical Education (CNME).[60] The AIH recognized the contributions of naturopathic physicians to the growth of the healing art by supporting the licensure of naturopathic physicians in all states; the existence of independent organizations to represent each licensed specialty; joint postgraduate educational programs; joint activities by all homeopathic professionals; the building of coalitions between homeopathy and other alternative groups outside the homeopathic community; a code of ethics for all homeopathic professionals; and collaboration in the creation of certification examinations.[61]

Not everyone applauded the inclusion of homeopathy in naturopathic medical education. Some wondered how different this was from the quasi-homeopathy that had been taught in the colleges during the nineteenth century. In fact, with the proliferation of questionable schools—some of which were blatant diploma mills offering their own self-authorized degrees—had the situation become even worse? Pseudo-homeopaths were stealing each other's intellectual property, advocating the virtues of polypharmacy, supporting frauds of multiple types, and advocating a "material miasm" of commercialism that tainted the school's history and accomplishments. American homeopaths, complained Greg Bedayn, RSHom, former editor of the *American Homeopath,* the journal of the North American Society of Homeopaths, seemed "to lack the ability to make a stand regarding the deceptions and charlatanism within our community, even when reliable principles for such a stand are close at hand." At issue was the lack of leadership and the unwillingness of anyone to take a stand in a climate dominated by political correctness. In essence, the issue was all about the failure of medical and professional ethics.[62]

In 1998, the Council on Homeopathic Education sent a questionnaire to all schools and institutions of classical homeopathy that operated in the United States and Canada. It represented the first attempt to assess the state of homeopathic training in North America in a "standardized" manner. From approximately thirty-six known schools, the council received only twenty-three replies.[63] Overall, the report suggested a wide diversity of practices, suggesting systemic problems in evaluation and program effectiveness. Of the twenty-three responding schools, the following information was obtained.

- Fourteen of the twenty-three schools were established in the 1990s; six in the 1980s; and two in the 1970s
- As of May 1998, there were 650 graduates of homeopathic programs that were either accredited or seeking accreditation
- Four of the schools had graduated between one and twenty students; five between twenty and fifty students; three between 50 and 100 students; and one more than 100 students
- Few of the schools had continued contact with their alumni after graduation and were therefore unable to report how many had become certified or were currently in practice
- Eighteen of the twenty-three schools focused solely on homeopathic training. The others offered homeopathy as a specialization or certificate within other degrees
- Thirteen of the twenty-three schools had obtained some level of governmental recognition
- Fourteen of the twenty-three schools were registered as non-profit organizations; eight were identified as for-profit entities
- Seven of the twenty-three schools identified themselves as post-graduate institutions designed for students with medical backgrounds
- Fourteen of the twenty-three schools offered graduate programs to students with medical training but without medical licenses; two of these schools were composed of more laypersons than students with medical training

- Six of the twenty-three institutions were located on the East Coast; eight on the West Coast; three in the Midwest; one in the South; and five in Canada
- Fourteen of the twenty-three institutions required at least one research project during the program; the remainder had no such requirement
- Library facilities were available in thirteen of the twenty-three institutions
- Three of the 23 institutions had only one professor; thirteen had between two and five; five had between six and nine; and two had ten or more teachers
- Twelve of the twenty-three institutions had advisory or governing boards
- Five of the twenty-three institutions had two-year programs; eight had three-year programs; and eight had four-year programs. An additional two had lengths ranging from summer school classes to six-month modules
- Actual class hours of homeopathic training ranged from 200 to 800 hours
- Student body size ranged from thirteen schools with fewer than fifty students; four between 50 and 150; and three with more than 150 students
- Thirteen of the twenty-three institutions limited class size to a maximum of forty students; six allowed between forty and sixty; and four allowed more than sixty students in lectures and discussions
- Six of the twenty-three institutions offered no clinical opportunities while seventeen offered at least limited supervision[64]

The evidence, sparse as it was since only twenty-three of the thirty-six known schools had responded, gave faint praise for what transpired as medical education. One can only imagine what Abraham Flexner would have written had he visited these schools or been privy to the responses in the questionnaires; and one can also imagine the feelings of former homeopathic faculty who had been roundly condemned as "mongrels" and "mixers" for their adjectival medicine.

For Joyce Frye, president of the AIH in 2004, the biggest issue in the homeopathic community was that of the unlicensed practitioner.

The public's perception of homeopathy encompassed all of its parts and, unfortunately, the perception it had of homeopathy was that of being "chaotic" and "unstructured." The issue surfaced at the June 2003 meeting of the Institute of Medicine Committee on Use of Complementary and Alternative Medicine. When asked what the AIH thought regarding licensure affecting the homeopathic profession, Frye responded that the AIH had no official position. However, on reflection, she thought the time had come "to put the moose on the table."[65]

Chapter 6

Whither the Future?

In its summer 2002 issue, the *American Journal of Homeopathic Medicine* (*AJHM*) published a series of articles highlighting a controversy involving the question of whether some reformers had gone too far in their acceptance of "new ideas" and thus undermined homeopathy by forsaking "disciplined thought and rational skepticism." The ideas in question included quantum theory, chaos theory, systems theory, and consciousness. Did these concepts alter the way homeopaths conducted provings? Did they change how homeopaths formulated ideas about the materia medica? Did they change how homeopaths administered their medicines?[1] Referenced in the exchange of views were the so-called essences of George Vithoulkas, the "physical pathology" encouraged by the Argentinian Francisco Xavier Eizayaga, and the later more subjective interpretations of symptoms, dreams, and correspondences with nature.[2] Many of these newer ideas were the work of well-known national and international teachers who reputedly had broken new ground in bridging Western and Eastern medicine and philosophy. This resulted in some homeopaths feeling the existence of a very real division emerging within classical homeopathy.

The "epicenter" for this discussion appeared in a series of letters and editorials emanating from an interview with George Vithoulkas that appeared in *Homeopathic Links* in 1999, a subsequent editorial by Julian Winston in *Homeopathy Today* in 2000, and an article in *Simillimum* in 2001 by Canadian naturopath André Saine. Winston criticized many of the speculative teachings of more recent homeopaths for going beyond the boundaries of classical homeopathy. Later in the same issue, he reviewed Nancy Herrick's book on animal provings and again cautioned against what he saw as too heavy a speculative character among the newer homeopaths.[3] Saine's article titled "Homeopathy versus Speculative Medicine: A Call to Action," accused Roger Morrison and his colleagues of prescribing "superficially," failing to teach the principles of the *Organon,* promoting speculative treatment, and spreading false doctrines.[4] For his part, Saine opposed those pseudo-homeopaths who practiced the doctrine of signatures; used remedies that conveyed themes, essences and central delusions; and employed new methodologies in case-taking, case analysis, and provings of medicines that were contrary to the principles of homeopathy enunciated by Hahnemann's. "The practice of medicine is sound as long as it is based on pure observation and correct reasoning," argued Saine. This was the "very heart of pure homeopathy" and was now being threatened by the teachings and practices of Morrison and his colleagues. All of the occult properties of plants that were subsumed into the doctrine of signatures had been rejected by Hahnemann. Thus to admit the doctrine into homeopathy was "not only a vain attempt at falsification of history but, even more grave, a misrepresentation of homeopathy."[5]

Saine went on to recount the speculative approach taken by Rajan Sankaran who had reported in *Homeopathic Links* the following:

> For many years I have advocated taking cases with virtually no questions. I believe that asking questions limits what we hear to only what we want to hear. In the process we lose the individuality of the patient and more often a more exact remedy.[6]

Here again, argued Saine, was a serious misrepresentation of Hahnemann's teachings. "Constant individualization is the trademark of pure homeopathy," he insisted, "while generalization is a consistent feature throughout conventional medicine. Medicine teaches that physicians who succeed in individualizing consequently succeed in curing, while the ones who generalize fail."[7] Those who committed errors of "generalization" and "poor methodology" were practicing the "antithesis of science and pure homeopathy."[8]

Saine, who was dean of the Canadian College of Homeopathy and editor of the works of Adolphe Lippe, expressed deep concern with beliefs and practices that were at variance with the principles of homeopathy and the scientific method. There were specified standards to which homeopaths must adhere to remain true to their science. Assuring this required peer review and constant watchfulness. For those who misrepresented homeopathy, he felt that their allegations and falsifications should be investigated and adjudicated by the profession.[9]

Saine identified ten of the most relevant principles of homeopathy.

1. The physician's main objective is to help the sick recover their health. . . . All personal ambitions and the desire to impress others must be set aside
2. The highest ideal of therapy is to restore health rapidly, gently, permanently; to remove and destroy the whole disease in the shortest, surest, least harmful way, according to clearly comprehensible principles
3. Medicines must first be proven on the healthy
4. The materia medica must be free from all speculation
5. The examination of the sick must be free from all speculation
6. The totality of the symptoms of the patient is the basis for choosing the most similar remedy. This means that the physician must conduct a thorough examination of the patient and gather all the subjective, objective, and circumstantial symptoms
7. The only medicinal disease agent meriting attention and preference in any case of disease is always the one that is most similar to the totality of the characteristic symptoms and that no petty bias should interfere with this serious choice
8. The remedy must be given singly, and in the optimal potency and repetition
9. The homeopathic physician constantly seeks to individualize the patient, the medicine, and its potency and repetition
10. Palliative treatments, regimens, or approaches are not compatible with the homeopathic treatment of patients presenting with curable dynamic diseases[10]

Quoting Hahnemann that "all conjecture, everything merely asserted or entirely fabricated must be completely excluded from such materia medica," Saine insisted that homeopathy, in its entirety, must be based on confirmed and reliable observation. Hahnemann insisted on mathematical certainty, not speculation; anything less was not true homeopathy.[11] Clearly, there were two different approaches to homeopathic medicine: one was Hahnemannian and the other non-Hahnemannian.

Unfortunately, many "pseudo-homeopaths" had chosen to identify themselves as Hahnemannians while, at the same time, misrepresenting the fundamental axioms of homeopathic medicine by failing to practice according to well-defined, clear principles. The difference was between deductive and inductive methods, and between a religious system built on belief and a science built on observation.[12]

Morrison, president of the Hahnemann Medical Clinic and instructor at Hahnemann College of Homeopathy, published his response in the Summer 2001 issue of *Homeopathy Today.* Supported by twenty-one colleagues, his response not only attempted to rebut Saine's accusations, but also called upon Winston to resign his editorship because of the "divisiveness" created by his editorial. Among the signers were Rajan Sankaran, Roger Jonathan Shore, Nancy Herrick, Corrie Hiwat, Harry van der Zee, and Deborah Collins.[13] Morrison took issue with the charges, repudiating Saine's claim that he and his colleagues had ventured beyond the principles of Hahnemann and were practicing "speculation" rather than good homeopathy. For Morrison, the idea of using the adaptive behaviors and habits of remedies was perfectly in keeping with Hahnemann's support and endorsement of experimentation. Thus, the observation that patients who required animal remedies were often consumed with thoughts of competition, that patients cured by snake venom showed "amazing similarity to snakes in their behavior," or that patients who used creeping plants and vines as remedies often produced dreams of traveling, seemed clearly to fall within mainstream homeopathy. In other words, "the true simillimum is imprinted on every aspect of the patient—his physical and mental symptoms, his dreams, his behavior."[14]

Although Morrison denied that either he or Sankaran adhered to the doctrine of signatures, his reasoning seemed weak at best, arguing that "the sources of our remedies do profoundly reflect themselves in the symptoms they produce." In other words, "the biology and adaptive behaviors of the plants and animals we utilize are imprinted upon the patient who needs the remedy." As for the accusation by Saine that he was developing a materia medica through cured cases instead of provings, Morrison responded hotly.

> [H]e does not acknowledge that the group of homeopaths he is criticizing (or excommunicating) have been among the most

> prolific provers of new remedies in the past hundred years. A single proving requires literally hundreds of man-hours. Imagine the predicament of myself and my colleagues: We are proving new remedies as fast as is humanly and responsibly possible while being taken to task by Crothers, Winston, Jacobs and others (none of whom have produced a single proving) for not doing a good enough job of it. On the other hand, when we reveal carefully devised strategies for prescribing poorly proved or little understood traditional remedies, we are equally reprimanded. Woe is me![15]

As the contentiousness spread, doctors Klaus Habich, Curt Kosters, and Jochen Rohwer weighed in on the side of Winston with the strong statement that the editor was "not alone in his criticism." Admitting that Morrison and the twenty-one signers of his letter were among homeopathy's predominant leaders, the question became just where did these leaders want to take homeopathy? What among their visionary ideas had anything to do with classical homeopathy?[16]

Among the items supported by Morrison and his colleagues as a source of homeopathic materia medica was the doctrine of signatures which, at the time of Hahnemann, inferred that the shape of a substance (i.e., bean) influenced the healer's ability to determine the organ the medicine was most likely to help (i.e., kidney). Hahnemann had rejected this doctrine as well as all other theoretical inferences—external and internal—that could not be directly deduced from observing the effects of the particular substance on the patient. For Hahnemann, each step had to be verifiable, which explained his emphasis on provings and extensive gathering of symptoms. Thus, wrote Habich and his co-authors, "anyone who deviates from the scientific mode of homeopathic practice . . . must be prepared for the inevitable question of what the deviation has to do with homeopathy." Between the symptoms of the patient and the remedy, they explained, the homeopath had to build a bridge of similars. Suggesting that the doctrine of signatures become a component of the homeopathic materia medica was significant, inasmuch as it violated the very foundations of homeopathic remedy research.[17]

There were limits, explained Habich, Kosters, and Rohwer, to what could be accepted as proof. If, for example, a minister of the interior chose to introduce visions as a form of evidence in a criminal procedure, society would quickly balk at the effort. Yet, here in medicine, certain homeopaths were not hesitating to prescribe remedies on the basis of a similar quality of evidence. At the very core of the debate, the critics argued, was the preservation of the materia medica. As for the doctrine of signatures (i.e., jealousy as a fundamental property of remedies of animal origin), it was "the abyss at the end of an inclined plane."[18]

> What right does someone have to claim he can draw inferences from the behavior of an animal as regards the medical efficacy of its milk? What makes people build complex structures of theory on the foundation of rubrics in the repertory when they have only to read about the symptoms in the primary literature to find out that it says something quite different there? When people begin to prove the Berlin Wall, at the latest, the whole thing becomes embarrassing. Once you get to magical thinking, it becomes quite arbitrary; for instance, should not differences be made between the wall in Berlin-Zehlendorf and Berlin-Kreuzberg? And what was the slogan written on the wall, anyway? And who was it written by? And why?[19]

In addition, Habich and his co-authors accused Dr. Mandanlal L. Sehgal and his supporters of using the repertory as a "magical object, as the soundboard of a cultural interpretation." While interesting, it was "certainly not science." Modern homeopathy, they explained, suffered from "sloppiness" of speculation. Homeopathy was not an "applied philosophy" or an "energetic or esoteric process"; rather it was the application of a healing technique "with a clear set of rules . . . as solid as those of mechanical engineering." If homeopathy was to remain a science, which the three critics clearly believed, then it had to adhere to "observable, explainable laws." This meant the ability to demonstrate remedy provings through the use of a double-blind test. For this to be so, homeopathy had to "free itself of scholastic thinking and find its way back to a scientific way of thinking."[20] For these critics, homeopathy led a "peripheral existence in science," teaching that which could be observed, but utilizing a potentization process that contradicted the paradigmatic foundation of the natural sciences.[21]

Dr. Richard Moskowitz, who had studied with both Vithoulkas and Sankaran, weighed in on the feud, lamenting what he considered was the end of an "era of good feelings" among homeopaths and a growing intolerance to innovative ideas from within the classical tradition. This included some of the most popular teachers—Rajan Sankaran, Jan Scholten, Massimo Mangialavori, Jeremy Sherr, and Nancy Herrick—whose ideas had been identified as "heretical and dangerous, or dismissed as frivolous and unworthy of serious consideration." Mediating between the opposing sides, Moskowitz noted that, with respect to the "essence" of a remedy, this concept had been controversial since its first introduction in the late nineteenth century. Nevertheless, the challenge of trying to look beyond the mass of symptoms to express or observe the drugs particular "genius" or "archetype" was something that all could appreciate. Certainly this had been the objective of Kent and his identification of the pulsatilla archetype. The remedy was not just "a mere assemblage of symptoms, but a living unity." However, Moskowitz cautioned that these archetypal essences or portraits depicted by Kent, Vithoulkas, Edward Whitmont, Catherine Coulter, Rajan Sankaran, and Jan Scholten were "never intended to circumvent or replace" more detailed study of remedies based on provings and clinical confirmations.[22]

A second theme in the new teachings stressed the mental and emotional symptoms that had also been championed by Kent and later elaborated by Whitmont, Vithoulkas, and Coulter. In Kent's *Lectures on Homeopathic Materia Medica* (1904) and Whitmont's *Psyche and Substance: Essays on Homeopathy in the Light of Jungian Psychology* (1982), the centerpiece of remedies was the mental and emotional characteristics with the physical symptoms in a secondary or ancillary grouping. In reflecting on his years as a practicing physician, J. H. Renner, MD, of California urged his fellow practitioners to let their hair down and discuss homeopathy "brutally and with frankness." For himself, he wondered if homeopathy had been "led astray" by the followers of Kent, thereby dissipating much of the heritage given by Hahnemann. Having spent untold hours over Kent's *Repertory,* Renner opined that Kent may have flown his kite too high.[23]

Moskowitz weighed in on this discussion as well, explaining that this had led to a "psychologizing tendency" by Sankaran where fears, dreams, and delusions merged with physical symptoms to reveal the patient's emotional state. This, in turn, had led to a reinterpretation of the totality of symptoms and the classification of remedies into kingdoms, plant and animal families, and mineral or chemical subgroups. While classical homeopathy had always assigned importance to highly subjective mental states, Moskowitz felt that Sankaran and his students had given them a higher priority, especially those derived from dreams, fears, and delusions. In fact, Sankaran went even further to focus on the collective unconscious and group dynamics, subjects never addressed by Hahnemann or any of the old masters in the field.[24]

A large part of what Moskowitz feared was the potential reincarnation of eclecticism and the "free-for-all atmosphere" that seemed to overtake homeopathy in the late nineteenth century. It was because of these tendencies that classical homeopathy had nearly died. Sensing that homeopathy's current revival was "still too new and too fragile to have sunk firm roots and developed stable traditions for the future," Moskowitz worried that the proliferation of teachers from many parts of the world offering seminars to anyone regardless of any prior homeopathic training was exposing homeopathy to danger. "Even for veteran prescribers," he observed, "the prevailing chaos fuels the need for readily identifiable standards."[25]

In an attempt to even out his criticism of the two opposing groups, Moskowitz accused Winston, Saine, Klaus-Henning Gypser, and Vithoulkas of "intemperate exaggeration" and "puritanical insistence on ideological purity." This "fundamentalist backlash" reminded him of Hahnemann's diatribe against the homeopaths of Leipzig whom he accused of treason and treachery. Moskowitz pointed out that Hahnemann himself had been a great innovator, as had been true of Kent and even Vithoulkas whose remedy "essences" had been dismissed by Kunzli and other physician-homeopaths as mere imagination. In retrospect, Moskowitz hoped that, notwithstanding the exaggerations and inaccuracies that accompanied the new thinkers, homeopaths would open themselves to this innovative generation of thinkers. "Disputes of this kind are a recurrent and indeed a central theme of our history," Moskowitz reasoned.

> They arise from the fact that homeopathy uniquely combines a practical method of healing the sick with a systematic philosophy of health and illness, that it calls for continual improvement

> and revision, yet rests on a conceptual framework that does not, cannot, and must not be allowed to change.

Both innovation and fundamentalism were vital parts of the definition of homeopathy.[26]

In reflecting on the controversy in a presentation before the Society of Homeopaths in the United Kingdom, Moskowitz reported that the dispute had become so contentious that old friendships had been broken and civility lost amid ideological differences. Characterizing the two opposing groups with the terms "innovation" and "fundamentalism," he noted that the first fundamentalist critique had come by way of Julian Winston's editorial in *Homeopathy Today* and represented the official view of the National Center for Homeopathy. His criticisms and those by Saine, Habich, and Jacobs which were directed at too much generalization and speculation, struck hard at the over mentalization of essences, signatures, and remedy families and kingdoms. What seemingly infuriated Moskowitz was the "Inquisitorial tone" of the accusers and their heavy-handed view of heresy as opposed to the possibility of "meaningful change" in the art of homeopathy. Moskowitz was particularly offended by their "Declaration of Principles" whose flavor was that of a loyalty oath followed by the threat of excommunication. For him, the "battle lines" had been drawn.[27]

Although not explicit in his comments, Moskowitz clearly viewed the fundamentalists as lacking in a full understanding and appreciation of homeopathy's long history. For in its past, each generation was marked by illustrative leaders whose writings and ideas stretched the genius of homeopathy's original leader. From Lippe to Kent to Vithoulkas, highly evocative ideas had surfaced to advance understanding between the individual proving symptoms and the patient. Thus Sankaran's quest to locate the dynamic core of the remedy was no more contrary or misleading or inaccurate than the essence of the remedy sought earlier by Kent and Vithoulkas. Moskowitz wrote:

> In our laudable zeal to defend the integrity and scientific rigor of his work, we often forget that Hahnemann, the fundamentalist *par excellence,* was also our greatest innovator . . . and maintained a lively curiosity about the science of his time, particularly in the "etheric" realms of clairvoyance, spiritualism, mesmerism, mediumship, and the like.

Thus, sitting in judgment rather than finding a middle ground between the innovators and fundamentalists seemed counterintuitive to the best interests of homeopathy. When Hahnemann railed against the "half-homeopaths" of Leipzig, he destroyed his own hope for a homeopathic hospital. As far as Moskowitz was concerned, the fundamentalists were committing the same error of judgment. "Homeopathy has . . . grown and developed over the years in important ways that the master did not and could not have foreseen, less by the addition of new remedies than in the depth of how we understand the ones we already know," he wrote. Better to see innovators and fundamentalists as "permanent features of our landscape," he advised, than to undermine the system with the forces of absolutism.[28]

Although Julian Winston had been party to the criticism as a result of his December 2000 editorial in *Homeopathy Today,* he also made an effort to calm both sides of the debate by suggesting that his editorial comments had been critical of both the right and left "edges" of homeopathy. "I was hoping that my comments might get people thinking about the vast grey area that defines what people call homeopathy," he wrote. "Instead, I was attacked on a personal level for daring to suggest that the people who used these methods are not homeopaths. I have always maintained that there are many ways to heal, homeopathy being just one modality." Time would tell if either of the "edges" had staying power.[29]

* * *

As one calculates the impact of homeopathy in the United States, it is difficult to ignore the internecine strife that seems perpetually to encompass and define this movement. Having successfully organized a strong and effective critique against orthodox medicine and having marshaled economic and political clout to establish an alternative structure of colleges, hospitals, and dispensaries to serve an appreciative public, homeopaths proceeded to advocate a host of metaphysical beliefs that, taken in the aggregate, split the movement between the extremes of low-potency adjuvant medicine at one end and high-potency mystical worldview at the other. Enthralled by a vision of a universe reduced to a single set of governing principles, homeopaths continue to articulate a philosophy that seems to satisfy their need for providential laws and purposes.

Nevertheless, homeopaths continue to be naïve in their conception of cause and effect, evasive of empirically based science, in denial as to the importance of controlled clinical trials, and blindly contemptuous of their encounter with the biomedical model. For better or worse, modern homeopathy invites comparison to some of the major religions in the world in that it seems capable of tolerating a multitude of dichotomies, pluralistic behaviors, fragmented discourses, and a penumbra of less than explicit healing therapies. Its growth and popularity are due less to the existence of a common creed than to a rapport for the primacy of spirit over matter, its attention to the restoration of harmony to the body's system, its metaphysical imagination, and unabashed openness to the acceptance of unseen forces. Whether homeopathy can survive as a belief system built on the undisciplined exaggerations and reinterpretations by nonmedically trained professionals remains to be seen. The beliefs and practices of modern homeopathy no longer stand on peer review and the scientific method. Instead, conjecture and open-ended speculation have trumped the fundamental axioms of homeopathic medicine and its once storied past.

Notes

Introduction

1. Andrew Weil, *Health and Healing* (Boston: Houghton Mifflin Company, 1983), 113-15.

2. See K. R. Pelletier, A. Marie, M. Krasner, and W. L. Haskell, "Current Trends in the Integration and Reimbursement of Complementary and Alternative Medicine by Managed Care, Insurance Carriers, and Hospital Providers," *American Journal of Health,* 12 (1997), 112-23; M. S. Wetzel, D. M. Eisenberg, and T. J. Kaptchuk, "A Survey of Courses Involving Complementary and Alternative Medicine in the United States Medical Schools," *Journal of the American Medical Association,* 280 (1998), 784-87; B. B. O'Connor, *Healing Traditions, Alternative Medicines and the Health Professions* (Philadelphia: University of Pennsylvania Press, 1995); D. M. Eisenberg, R. C. Kessler, C. Foster, et al., "Unconventional Medicine in the United States—Prevalence, Costs, and Patterns of Use," *New England Journal of Medicine,* 328 (1993), 246-52; J. A. Astin, "Why Patients Use Alternative Medicines," *Journal of the American Medical Association,* 279 (1998), 1548-53; Mike Saks, "Medicine and the Counter Culture," in Roger Cooter and John Pictstone (eds.), *Medicine in the Twentieth Century* (Australia: Harwood Academic Publishers, 2000), 122.

Chapter 1

1. Daniel Cook and Alain Naudé, "The Ascendance and Decline of Homeopathy in America: How Great Was Its Fall?" *Journal of the American Institute of Homeopathy,* 89 (1996), 126-39. See also Anne T. Korschman, "Making Friends for 'Pure' Homeopathy: Hahnemannianism and the Twentieth Century Preservation and Transformation of Homeopathy," in Robert D. Johnston (ed.), *The Politics of Healing* (New York: Routledge, 2004), 29-53.

2. Julian Winston, "Keeping It Alive: Homeopathy Through the First Half of the Century," *Journal of the American Institute of Homeopathy,* 92 (1999), 215-16. See also John S. Haller, Jr., *A Profile in Alternative Medicine: The Eclectic Medical College of Cincinnati, 1845-1942* (Kent, Ohio: Kent State University Press, 1999), 79-82; Julian Winston, *The Faces of Homeopathy: An Illustrated History of the First 200 Years* (Tawa, New Zealand: Great Auk Publishers, 1999), 226-29.

3. Winston, "Keeping it Alive: Homeopathy Through the First Half of the Century," 217.

4. "Minutes of the Sixty-Eighth Session," *Journal of the American Institute of Homeopathy,* 5 (1912-13), 166.

5. Stuart M. Close, "A Century of Homeopathy in America," *Homeopathic Recorder,* 40 (1925), 509.

6. Alonzo C. Tenney, "Homeopathy," *Journal of the American Institute of Homeopathy,* 4 (1911), 35-38.

7. Close, "A Century of Homeopathy in America," 513.

8. Quoted in Henry D. Paine, "Proceedings of Societies," *American Homeopathic Review,* 1 (1859), 467-68.

9. Quoted in Bushrod W. James, "History of the American Institute of Homeopathy," *Homeopathic Recorder,* 17 (1902), 248-49. See also Carroll Dunham, *Homeopathy, the Science of Therapeutics: A Collection of Papers Elucidating and Illustrating the Principles of Homeopathy* (Calcutta: Haren and Brother, 1973).

10. Quoted in Charles Francis Ring, "Some Thoughts on a New Remedial Source," *Homeopathic Recorder,* 2 (1887), 7.

11. Arthur G. Allen, "Specialties, from a Homeopathic Standpoint," *Medical Advance,* 22 (1889), 366-67.

12. Interestingly, the International Hahnemannian Association faced its own schism in 1895 when a group of Hahnemannians decided that the association was not pure enough and split off forming the Society of Homeopathicians. See Martin Kaufman, *Homeopathy in America: The Rise and Fall of a Medical Heresy* (Baltimore: Johns Hopkins University Press, 1971), 121.

13. Plumb Brown, "The President's Message," *Homeopathic Recorder,* 46 (1931), 549.

14. A. G. Allen, "Post-Graduate School of Homeopathics," *Medical Advance,* 27 (1891), 371-74.

15. "Editorial," *Medical Advance,* 37 (1900), 345-46. See also Winston, *The Faces of Homeopathy,* 528-33.

16. "Miscellany," *Medical Advance,* 30 (1893), 26.

17. "Annual Announcement, 1901-1902," *Medical Advance,* 39 (1901), 339, 342-43; "Hering Medical College Department," *Medical Advance,* 37 (1899), 206-207.

18. "Homeopathic Retrogression," *Homeopathic Recorder,* 35 (1920), 575-76.

19. "The Organization of Three State Boards of Medical Examiners Under the New York Law of 1890," *Medical Advance,* 27 (1891), 133.

20. J. A. Streets, "Medical Legislation," *Medical Advance,* 23 (1889), 9-11.

21. C. E. Walton, "Presidential Address: Ohio State Society," *Medical Advance,* 23 (1889), 15.

22. H. M. Paine, "New York Medical Examiners," *Medical Advance,* 27 (1891), 135-36.

23. "The American Institute of Homeopathy," *Medical Advance,* 39 (1901), 324-25.

24. Harvey Farrington, "Symptomatic versus Pathologic Prescribing," *Journal of the American Institute of Homeopathy,* 34 (1941), 586. See also Harris L. Coulter, *Divided Legacy: A History of the Schism in Medical Thought. Vol. III. Science and Ethics in American Medicine, 1800-1914* (Washington, D.C.: Wehawken Book Co., 1977), 328-401.

25. William L. Morgan, "How to Train a Physician to Practice Homeopathy," *Homeopathic Recorder,* 18 (1903), 433-34.

26. "Adjectival Homeopathy," *Medical Advance,* 41 (1903), 358-60.

27. Stuart M. Close, "The Hahnemannian as a Specialist," *Medical Advance,* 42 (1904), 671-77.

28. Old Timer, "The New Homeopathy," *Homeopathic Recorder,* 19 (1904), 260.

29. Morgan, "How to Train a Physician to Practice Homeopathy," 434.

30. Morgan, "How to Train a Physician to Practice Homeopathy," 436-39.

31. Robert Hudson, "Abraham Flexner in Perspective: American Medical Education, 1865-1910," *Bulletin of the History of Medicine,* 46 (1972), 545-61; Howard S. Berliner, "A Larger Perspective on the Flexner Report," *International Journal of Health Sciences,* 5 (1975), 573-92.

32. Abraham Flexner, *Medical Education in the United States and Canada; A Report of the Carnegie Foundation for the Advancement of Teaching* (New York: Carnegie Foundation for the Advancement of Teaching, 1910), 159-61.

33. George Royal, "The Art and Science of Medicine," *Journal of the American Institute of Homeopathy,* 3 (1910), 301-302.

34. "Massachusetts," *Journal of the American Institute of Homeopathy,* 3 (1910), 434. See also "The Carnegie Report and Boston University," *New England Medical Gazette,* 45 (1910), 372-73.

35. Royal, "Editorial," *Journal of the American Institute of Homeopathy,* 3 (1910), 751.

36. "Report of the Council of Medical Education," *Journal of the American Institute of Homeopathy,* I (1909), 361.

37. "The Hahnemann Medical College of Philadelphia," *Journal of the American Institute of Homeopathy,* 3 (1910), 289.

38. Willis Alonzo, "Medical Education in the Homeopathic School of Medicine," *Report, U.S. Bureau of Education,* I (1914), 219-22.

39. Stuart M. Close, "Compensating Correspondence," *Homeopathic Recorder,* 40 (1925), 273-76.

40. "Homeopathic Organizations in the United States," *Journal of the American Institute of Homeopathy,* 4 (1912), 1123-24.

41. Scott Parsons, "Business Session of AIH," *Journal of the American Institute of Homeopathy,* 9 (1916-17), 328-29.

42. G. M. Cushing, "Taking Stock of Our Homeopathic Colleges," *Journal of the American Institute of Homeopathy,* 11 (1918-19), 89-90. See also Harris L. Coulter, *Divided Legacy: A History of the Schism in Medical Thought. Vol. III. Science and Ethics in American Medicine, 1800-1914* (Washington, D.C.: Wehawken Book Co., 1977), 446-47.

43. "Editorial," *Journal of the American Institute of Homeopathy,* 11 (1918-19), 581-82.

44. James W. Ward, "University of California: Report of the Committee on Homeopathic Instruction," *Journal of the American Institute of Homeopathy,* 12 (1919-20), 367-70.

45. "Department of Homeopathic Materia Medica and Therapeutics in the College of Medicine of the State University of Iowa," *Journal of the American Institute*

of Homeopathy, 11 (1918-19), 1302; S. Persons, "The Decline of Homeopathy—The University of Iowa, 1876-1919," *Bulletin of the History of Medicine,* 65 (1991), 79-82.

46. Thomas J. Preston, "The College Situation and Prospects," *Journal of the American Institute of Homeopathy,* 12 (1919-20), 473, 477.

47. Claude A. Burnett, "Modern Medical Education," *Journal of the American Institute of Homeopathy,* 13 (1920-21), 150.

48. "The University of Michigan Homeopathic Medical School," *Journal of the American Institute of Homeopathy,* 14 (1921-22), 550-54; "Special Meeting of the Michigan Society," *Journal of the American Institute of Homeopathy,* 14 (1921-22), 665; "Contributed Editorial: The Michigan Merger," *Journal of the American Institute of Homeopathy,* 14 (1921-22), 702-703.

49. "Summer Course in Homeopathy at Michigan," *Journal of the American Institute of Homeopathy,* 15 (1922-23), 961-62.

50. "A Tribute," *Journal of the American Institute of Homeopathy,* 15 (1922-23), 401; W. H. Roberts, "Orthodoxy vs. Homeopathy: Ironic Developments Following the Flexner Report of the Ohio State University," *Bulletin of the History of Medicine,* 60 (1986), 73-87.

51. "Hahnemann of Chicago Reorganized," *Journal of the American Institute of Homeopathy,* 15 (1922-23), 179.

52. "Report of the Council on Medical Education," *Journal of the American Institute of Homeopathy,* 15 (1922-23), 251-52.

53. "Where Shall I Study Medicine?" *Journal of the American Institute of Homeopathy,* 15 (1922-23), 686-87.

54. "Homeopathy—A Review of Its Condition at the Present Time," *Homeopathic Recorder,* 35 (1920), 239-40.

55. Rudolph F. Rabe, "The Perpetuation of Homeopathy," *Journal of the American Institute of Homeopathy,* 32 (1939), 237-39.

56. Conrad Wesselhoeft, "Elementary Homeopathy," *Journal of the American Institute of Homeopathy,* 20 (1927), 105-107, 119.

57. Dr. August Bier, "What Shall Be Our Attitude Toward Homeopathy?" *Homeopathic Recorder,* 40 (1925), 562-63.

58. E. Wallace MacAdam, "Homeopathic Tides," *Journal of the American Institute of Homeopathy,* 21 (1928), 204-206.

59. Linn J. Boyd, "What is Essential?" *Journal of the American Institute of Homeopathy,* 20 (1927), 864-70.

60. Linn J. Boyd, "Some Factors Responsible for the Recent Progress in Homeopathy," *Journal of the American Institute of Homeopathy,* 24 (1931), 1222-24.

61. H. Wapler, "The Incorporation of Homeopathy into United Medicine," *Journal of the American Institute of Homeopathy,* 25 (1932), 3-11.

62. Wapler, "The Incorporation of Homeopathy into United Medicine," 3-11.

63. John P. Sutherland, "Homeopathy from the Standpoint of Evolution," *Journal of the American Institute of Homeopathy,* 21 (1928), 770-71.

64. John B. Sutherland, "Progressive Homeopathy," *Journal of the American Institute of Homeopathy,* 23 (1930), 74-75.

65. "Sectarianism and Dogmatism," *Journal of the American Institute of Homeopathy,* 29 (1936), 116-17.

66. J. C. Hayner, "Acerbity," *Journal of the American Institute of Homeopathy,* 29 (1936), 247-48.

67. Harold R. Griffith, "The Field of Homeopathic Remedies in Scientific Medicine," *Journal of the American Institute of Homeopathy,* 23 (1930), 764.

68. "Some Causes of Disintegration," *Homeopathic Recorder,* 37 (1922), 427-29.

69. Stuart M. Close, "Progress in Medicine and the Amplified Totality," *Homeopathic Recorder,* 37 (1922), 469-71. See also Coulter, *Divided Legacy: A History of the Schism in Medical Thought. Vol. III. Science and Ethics in American Medicine, 1800-1914,* 443-44.

70. Alfred Pulford, "Sold Out," *Homeopathic Recorder,* 37 (1922), 458-61.

71. Rudolph F. Rabe, "Some Reminiscences of a Homeopathic Physician," *Homeopathic Recorder,* 47 (1932), 554.

72. Rudolph F. Rabe, "Defining the Sphere of Homeopathy," *Journal of the American Institute of Homeopathy,* 36 (1943), 169-70.

73. Donald A. Davis, "The Viewpoint of the Younger Generation Regarding Homeopathy," *Homeopathic Recorder,* 52 (1937), 177.

74. Stuart M. Close, "The Pendulum of Progress—A New Year Meditation," *Homeopathic Recorder,* 40 (1925), 29-30, 33-34.

75. Close, "A Century of Homeopathy in America," *Homeopathic Recorder,* 40 (1925), 505.

76. Stuart Close, "Homeopathic Philosophy and Modern Medicine," *Homeopathic Recorder,* 41 (1926), 167.

77. Close, "Homeopathic Philosophy and Modern Medicine," 168, 173.

78. Stuart Close, "Medical Protestantism," *Homeopathic Recorder,* 42 (1927), 422-23.

79. Close, "Homeopathic Philosophy and Modern Medicine," 174-76.

80. Stuart Close, "Incentives to Industry in Homeopathy," *Homeopathic Recorder,* 40 (1925), 416-18.

81. Close, "Incentives to Industry in Homeopathy," 418-19.

82. "Resolutions Pertaining to Rating of Homeopathic Colleges," *Journal of the American Institute of Homeopathy,* 29 (1936), 44-45.

83. "A Right Time and a Wrong Time for Criticism," *Journal of the American Institute for Homeopathy,* 29 (1936), 314. See also Naomi Rogers, "The Proper Place of Homeopathy: Hahnemannian Medical College and Hospital in an Age of Scientific Medicine," *Pennsylvania Magazine of History and Biography,* 108 (1984), 179-201.

84. A. W. Records, "Meeting of the Congress of States, Palmer House, Chicago," *Journal of the American Institute of Homeopathy,* 29 (1936), 251.

85. E. Wallace MacAdam and William Gutman, "Homeopathic News," *Journal of the American Institute of Homeopathy,* 41 (1948), 181.

86. Records, "Meeting of the Congress of States, Palmer House, Chicago," 251-52.

87. E. B. J., "The Status of Homeopathy," *Journal of the American Institute of Homeopathy,* 32 (1939), 90. See Also Naomi Rogers, *An Alternative Path: The*

Making and Remaking of Hahnemann Medical College and Hospital of Philadelphia (New Brunswick: Rutgers University Press, 1998).

88. William Wallace Young, "A Review of the Status of Homeopathic Education in the United States of America," *Journal of the American Institute of Homeopathy,* 39 (1946), 108; Charles L. Brown, "Homeopathic Education," *Journal of the American Institute of Homeopathy,* 40 (1947), 112; Willis A. Dewey, "History of Homeopathy in California," *Pacific Coast Journal of Homeopathy,* 50 (1939), 219-24.

89. Claude A. Burnett, "Medical Education," *Journal of the American Institute of Homeopathy,* 26 (1933), 600. See also Andrew Cunningham and Perry Williams (eds.), *The Laboratory Revolution in Medicine* (New York: Cambridge University Press, 1992).

90. Rudolph F. Rabe, "Is Homeopathic Practice Threatened with Extinction," *Journal of the American Institute of Homeopathy,* 44 (1951), 276-77.

91. Winston, "Keeping It Alive: Homeopathy Through the First Half of the Century," 221-23.

Chapter 2

1. See Rudi Verspoor and Steven Decker, *Homeopathy Re-Examined—Beyond the Classical Paradigm* (Ontario, Canada: Hahnemann Center for Heilkunst, 1999). The authors suggest that so-called classical homeopathy has a flawed lineage due in large measure to poor translations of Hahnemann's works and the consequence of his philosophy being distorted among many supporters. See also Anthony Campbell, *The Two Faces of Homeopathy* (London: R. Hale, 1984); Martin Dinges, "The Contribution of the Comparative Approach to the History of Homeopathy," in Robert Jütte, Motzi Eklöf, and Marie C. Nelson (eds.), *Historical Aspects of Unconventional Medicine* (Sheffield: EAHMH, 2001), 51-72.

2. See Matthew Wood, *The Magical Staff: The Vitalist Tradition in Western Medicine* (Berkeley: North Atlantic, 1992); Leonard Richmond Wheeler, *Vitalism: Its History and Validity* (London: H.F. and G. Witherby, 1939); Marc C. Micozzi, *Fundamentals of Complementary and Alternative Medicine* (New York: Churchill Livingston, 2001), 43-56.

3. "Theory of Life," *American Homeopathic Review,* I (1858), 49-50, 97-101.

4. "Theory of Cure," *American Homeopathic Review,* II (1859), 106, 145.

5. "Theory of Cure," 146-49.

6. Rufus Choate, "How do Medicines Act?" *Homeopathic Recorder,* 3 (1888), 57-58.

7. Roger G. Perkins, "Remedies," *American Homeopathic Review,* I (1859), 388.

8. C. J. Hempel, "Lehrbuch Der Homeopathie by Dr. V. Grauvogl," *American Homeopathic Observer,* 7 (1870), 361-62.

9. Quoted in Benjamin C. Woodbury, "Homeopathy and the New Vitalism," *Homeopathic Recorder,* 43 (1928), 128.

10. Woodbury, "Homeopathy and the New Vitalism," 131-32, 136.

11. Francis Trueherz, "The Origins of Kent's Homeopathy," *Journal of the American Institute of Homeopathy,* 77 (1984), 130-49; Harold Gardiner, "Swedenborg's Philosophy and Modern Science," *British Homeopathic Journal,* 49 (1960), 195; Scott Trego Swank, *The Unfettered Conscience, A Study of Sectarianism, Spiritualism and Social Reform in the New Jerusalem Church* (PhD Dissertation, University of Pennsylvania, 1970); Clement John Wilkinson, *John James Garth Wilkinson. A Memoir of His Life with a Selection from His Letters* (London: Kegan Paul Trench Trubner, 1911); Richard De Charms, *Hahnemann and Swedenborg; Or the Affinities Between the Fundamental Principles of Homeopathia and the Doctrines of the New Church* (Philadelphia: New Jerusalem Printers, 1850).

12. Hempel, "Lehrbuch Der Homeopathie by Dr. V. Grauvogl," 365-67, 371-72.

13. W. L. Morgan, "Five Distinctive Principles of Homeopathy," *Homeopathic Recorder,* 19 (1904), 356-57.

14. "New Publications," *Homeopathic Recorder,* 3 (1888), 128-30.

15. Charles L. Olds, "Life and Vital Force," *Homeopathic Recorder,* 46 (1931), 783. See also Robert C. Fuller, *Alternative Medicine and American Religious Life* (New York: Oxford University Press, 1989); Elinore Peebles, "Homeopathy and the New Church," in Robin Larsen (ed.), *Emanuel Swedenborg: A Continuing Vision* (New York: Swedenborg Foundation, 1988), 468-72.

16. See John S. Haller, Jr., *The History of American Homeopathy: The Academic Years, 1820-1936* (Binghamton, New York: Haworth Press Inc., 2005), 236-42; Frank Trueherz, "The Origins of Kent's Homeopathy," *Journal of the American Institute of Homeopathy,* 77 (1984), 130-49; Wood, *The Magical Staff,* Julian Winston, *The Faces of Homeopathy: An Illustrated History of the First 200 Years* (Tawa, New Zealand: Great Awk Publishers, 1999), 166-67.

17. James Tyler Kent, *Repertory of the Homeopathic Materia Medica* (New Delhi: World Homeopathic Links, 1982), xix. See also E. Van Galen, "Kent's Hidden Links: The Influence of Emanuel Swedenborg on the Homeopathic Philosophy of James Tyler Kent," *Homeopathic Links,* 7 (1994), 27-39; 37-38.

18. Peter Morrell, "Kent's Influence on British Homeopathy," *Journal of the American Institute of Homeopathy,* 92 (1999-2000), 228.

19. James Tyler Kent, *New Remedies, Clinical Cases, Lesser Writings, Aphorisms and Precepts* (Chicago: Ehrhart and Karl, 1926), 97.

20. John P. Sutherland, "Boston University School of Medicine: Address at the Opening of the 47th Annual Session," *Journal of the American Institute of Homeopathy,* 12 (1919-20), 716-17.

21. Olds, "Life and Vital Force," 782, 791.

22. "Faith versus Knowledge," *Medical Advance,* 23 (1889), 193-94.

23. Stuart Close, "Coordinating Theology with Medicine," *Homeopathic Recorder,* 41 (1926), 323-24, 326-27.

24. Benjamin C. Woodbury, "Orientation in Homoeopathy," *Homeopathic Recorder,* 26 (1921), 454, 528-29.

25. Woodbury, "Orientation in Homoeopathy," 531-32, 542-53.

26. Alfred Pulford, "The Cure and Prevention of Disease," *Homeopathic Recorder,* 36 (1921), 442-43.

27. Stuart M. Close, "General Interpretations in Science and Philosophy," *Homeopathic Recorder,* 35 (1920), 178-81. See also A. Wilford Hall, *The Problem of Human Life* (New York: Hall and Company, 1877).

28. Stuart Close, "The Identity of Hahnemann's 'Vital Force' with the Subconscious Mind," *Homeopathic Recorder,* 38 (1923), 312-13, 316, 320-21.

29. Dr. Pierre Schmidt, "Homeopathic Education," *Homeopathic Recorder,* 40 (1925), 433-36.

30. Dr. Dudgeon, "How Hahnemann Cured," *Homeopathic Recorder,* 5 (1890), 215-19.

31. Dr. C. Von Boenninghausen, "Articles by Dr. C. V. Boenninghausen. The Value of High Potencies," *Homeopathic Recorder,* 22 (1907), 154-55. See also Bernhardt Fincke, *On High Potencies and Homeopathics* (Philadelphia: A. J. Tafel, 1865).

32. Dudgeon, "How Hahnemann Cured," 220-21. See also George F. Foote, *Dr. Foote's Potentizer* (n.p.: Hoyne, 1854).

33. "Potency," *Homeopathic Recorder,* 4 (1889), 241-43.

34. Quoted in J. H. Holloway, "The Material and the Immaterial Dose," *Homeopathic Recorder,* 26 (1911), 154.

35. Holloway, "The Material and Immaterial Dose," 154, 156.

36. John Prentice Rand, "The Theory of Dynamization, Is It Scientifically Tenable?" *Journal of the American Institute of Homeopathy,* 5 (1912-13), 555-56.

37. Benjamin C. Woodbury and Harry B. Baker, "Testing the Potentiality of Drugs," *Homeopathic Recorder,* 37 (1922), 529, 531-32.

38. Woodbury and Baker, "Testing the Potentiality of Drugs," 534-35, 541.

39. F. K. Bellokossy, "X-Ray Potencies," *Journal of the American Institute of Homeopathy,* 40 (1947), 160-62.

40. Federico Anaya-Reyes, "X-Ray and Its Application According to Homeopathy and the Law of Arndt-Schulz," *Journal of the American Institute of Homeopathy,* 58 (1965), 24-25.

41. "The Twelve Tissue Remedies of Schüssler," *Homeopathic Recorder,* 14 (1899), 274. See also Constantine Hering, *The Twelve Tissue Remedies and Their Use in Trituration of Dr. Schüssler* (New York: Boericke and Tafel, 1874).

42. F. E. Stoaks, "The Tissue Remedies and Their Relation to Homeopathy," *Homeopathic Recorder,* 9 (1894), 391-93.

43. "Notes," *Homeopathic Recorder,* 9 (1894), 568. See also William Boericke and Willis A. Dewey, *The Twelve Tissue Remedies of Schüssler* (Philadelphia: Boericke and Tafel, 1893).

44. Quoted in Leon Renard, "Concerning Schüssler's Twelve Remedies," *Journal of the American Institute of Homeopathy,* 33 (1940), 365.

45. Eric Vondergoltz, "The Relation Between Hahnemann and Schüssler," *Homeopathic Recorder,* 18 (1903), 109-115.

46. Renard, "Concerning Schüssler's Twelve Remedies," 366.

47. André Saine, "Fads, Trends, and Dogma Undermining the Quality of the Practice of Homeopathy in America," *Journal of the American Institute of Homeopathy,* 87 (1994) 196-98; Trevor M. Cook, *Homeopathic Medicine Today* (New Canaan, Connecticut: Keats Publishing, Inc., 1989), 42-43.

48. Quoted in Mechthild Scheffer, *Bach Flower Therapy: Theory and Practice* (Rochester, Vermont: Healing Arts Press, 1988), 13.

49. Cook, *Homeopathic Medicine Today,* 43.

50. See Jeffrey G. Shapiro, *The Flower Remedy Book* (Berkeley: North Atlantic Books, 1999); Julian Barnard, *Bach Flower Remedies; Form and Function* (Massachusetts: Lindisfarne Books, 2004); C. G. Harvey and A. Cochrane, *The Encyclopaedia of Flower Remedies* (London: Thorson's, 1995); P. Mansfield, *Flower Remedies* (London: Optima, 1995); Steven B. Kayne, *Complementary Therapies for Pharmacists* (London: Pharmaceutical Press, 2002), 245-51.

51. Stuart M. Close, "The Development of Hahnemannian Philosophy in the Sixth Edition of the *Organon,*" *Homeopathic Recorder,* 38 (1923), 507-511.

52. "Hahnemann's *Organon,* Sixth Edition," *Homeopathic Recorder,* 37 (1922), 239.

53. Stuart M. Close, "A Century of Homeopathy in America," *Homeopathic Recorder,* 40 (1925), 516.

54. Woodbury and Baker, "Testing the Potentiality of Drugs," 481-85.

55. Dr. Kirn, "Homeopathy and the 'OD' Theory," *Homeopathic Recorder,* 42 (1927), 529-41. See also Robert Rohland, *Od, or Odo-Magnetic, Force: An Explanation of Its Influence on Homeopathic Medicines, from the Odic Point of View* (New York: n.p., 1871).

56. Guy Beckley Stearns, "Physics of High Dilutions," *Homeopathic Recorder,* 46 (1931), 400. See also Albert Abrams, *New Concepts in Diagnosis and Treatment* (San Francisco: Philopolis Press, 1916).

57. Benjamin C. Woodbury, "Homeopathic Attenuations and the Electronic Reactions of Abrams," *Homeopathic Recorder,* 35 (1920), 53-57.

58. [Committee Report], *Homeopathic Recorder,* 35 (1923), 443-45.

59. Stearns, "Physics of High Dilutions," 401.

60. "The American Institute of Homeopathy and the Abrams Theory," *Journal of the American Institute of Homeopathy,* 16 (1923), 190.

61. "Foundation for Homeopathic Research," *Journal of the American Institute of Homeopathy,* 15 (1922-23), 1015.

62. Stearns, "Physics of High Dilutions," 398-99.

63. Sir John Weir, "Present Day Confirmation of Homeopathy," *Journal of the American Institute of Homeopathy,* 48 (1955), 375. See also W. E. Boyd, *Research on the Low Potencies of Homeopathy* (London: William Heinemann, 1936); W. Ritchie McCrae, "Our Debt to the Late Dr. W. E. Boyd and the British Homeopathic Association," *The Layman Speaks,* 9 (1956), 7-9.

64. "Homeopathy Abroad," *The Layman Speaks,* 15 (1961), 159.

65. J. L. Kaplowe, "Science and Homeopathy," *Homeopathic Recorder,* 53 (1937), 492-93. See also Herbert A. Roberts, *The Principles and Art of Cure by Homeopathy* (Halsworthy, England: Health Science Press, 1942).

66. Harvey Farrington, "Curantur vs. Curentur," *Homeopathic Recorder,* 50 (1935), 129-31.

67. E. G. H. Miessler, "Curantur, Curentur, Curenter," *Homeopathic Recorder,* 15 (1900), 25-27.

68. E. G. H. Miessler, "Dr. E. G. H. M. Again Says Curantur," *Homeopathic Recorder,* 15 (1900), 400-403.

69. "Curantur or Curentur," *Journal of the American Institute of Homeopathy,* 26 (1933), 591.

70. E. G. H. Miessler, "Curentur Wrong from the Grammatical Point of View," *Homeopathic Recorder,* 16 (1901), 32-33.

71. "Constitution and By-Laws," *Journal of the American Institute of Homeopathy,* 4 (1912), 1487.

72. G. H. Thacher, "What is the Difference?" *Homeopathic Recorder,* 43 (1928), 88.

73. Farrington, "Curantur vs. Curentur," 129-31.

74. "Editorial," *Journal of American Institute of Homeopathy,* 81 (1988), 57-58; Peter Fisher, "Letter to the Editor," *Journal of the American Institute of Homeopathy,* 81 (1988), 61.

75. Randall Neustaedter, "Law of Similars II," *Journal of the American Institute of Homeopathy,* 81 (1988), 66-69.

76. Harris Coulter, "Law of Similars III," *Journal of the American Institute of Homeopathy,* 81 (1988), 70-71.

77. William Shevin, "Law of Similars IV," *Journal of the American Institute of Homeopathy,* 81 (1988), 72-73.

78. Ahmed Currim, "Similia Similibus Curentur: A Natural Law," *Journal of the American Institute of Homeopathy,* 81 (1988), 94-99.

79. Richard Moskowitz, "More on Similia Similibus Curentur," *Journal of the American Institute of Homeopathy,* 81 (1988), 139-41.

80. "Esoteric Homeopathy," *Homeopathic Recorder,* 40 (1925), 376-77.

Chapter 3

1. Julia M. Green, "American Foundation for Homeopathy," *Homeopathic Recorder,* 37 (1922), 557-58. See Ann Taylor Kirschman, "Struggle for Survival: The American Foundation for Homeopathy and the Preservation of Homeopathy in the United States, 1920-1930," in Martin Dinges (ed.), *Patients in the History of Homeopathy* (Sheffield: EAHMHP, 2002), 373-90.

2. Julia M. Green, "Homeopathy Optimistic," *Journal of the American Institute of Homeopathy,* 20 (1927), 421-23.

3. Julia M. Green, "The Outlook for Homeopathy," *Homeopathic Recorder,* 43 (1928), 7-9.

4. "Salute to a Veteran," *Journal of the American Institute of Homeopathy,* 57 (1964), 58.

5. H. A. Roberts, "Post-Graduate School of the American Foundation for Homeopathy," *Homeopathic Recorder,* 47 (1932), 361-63.

6. "Editorial," *Homeopathic Recorder,* 51 (1936), 470-78.

7. Julia M. Green, "Report of the Board of Medical Education," *Journal of the American Institute of Homeopathy,* 43 (1950), 210-11.

8. Carl H. Enstam, "Postgraduate Homeopathic Education on the Pacific Coast," *Journal of the American Institute of Homeopathy,* 40 (1947), 167-68.

9. William Wallace Young, "A Review of the Status of Homeopathic Education in the United States of America," *Journal of the American Institute of Homeopathy,* 39 (1946), 108.

10. Victor C. Laughlin, "Practical Steps in Homeopathic Postgraduate Education," *Journal of the American Institute of Homeopathy,* 40 (1947), 165-66.

11. George Royal, "World Progress in Homeopathy," *Journal of the American Institute of Homeopathy,* 23 (1930), 79-83.

12. Ray W. Spalding, "A Postgraduate Teaching Program," *Journal of the American Institute of Homeopathy,* 43 (1950), 97.

13. "A Prevailing Question," *Journal of the American Institute of Homeopathy,* 32 (1939), 754.

14. Julia M. Green, "Postgraduate Instruction in the Future of Homeopathy," *Journal of the American Institute of Homeopathy,* 39 (1946), 331.

15. "The Foundation Postgraduate Course," *Journal of the American Institute of Homeopathy,* 48 (1955), 219-20.

16. Michael R. Romaner, "A Layman's Observations," *The Layman Speaks,* 28 (1975), 223-25.

17. Stuart M. Close, "Educating the Layman," *Homeopathic Recorder,* 37 (1922), 512-17.

18. James Krauss, "The Definition of Medicine," *Journal of the American Institute of Homeopathy,* 4 (1911), 339-41.

19. Green, "American Foundation for Homeopathy," 558-59. See also Julian Winston, *The Faces of Homeopathy: An Illustrated History of the First 200 Years* (Tawa, New Zealand: Great Awk Publishers, 1999), 346-47; Anne Taylor Kirschman, "Making Friends for 'Pure' Homeopathy: Hahnemannians and the Twentieth Century Preservation and Transformation of Homeopathy," in Robert D. Johnston (ed.), *The Politics of Healing* (New York: Routledge, 2004), 29-42.

20. "Laymen's Leagues," *Homeopathic Recorder,* 38 (1923), xvii-xviii.

21. "Laymen's Leagues Under the American Foundation for Homeopathy Bureau of Publicity," *Journal of the American Institute of Homeopathy,* 36 (1943), 24-25.

22. Elizabeth Stuart Close, "The Laymen's Plea," *Journal of the American Institute of Homeopathy,* 37 (1944), 28.

23. Max Shernoff, "A Layman's Experience with Homeopathy," *Journal of the American Institute of Homeopathy,* 40 (1947), 102-104.

24. J. W. Waffensmith, "The Rising Voice of the Laymen," *Journal of the American Institute of Homeopathy,* 37 (1944), 101-102.

25. "Accomplishments of the AIH," *Homeopathic Recorder,* 41 (1926), xi-xxiii.

26. "Down to Bed Rock," *Journal of the American Institute of Homeopathy,* 28 (1935), 170-71. See also Winston, *The Faces of Homeopathy,* 398-401.

27. A. W. Belting, "Our Educational Duties and Plans from the Standpoint of the Laity," *Journal of the American Institute of Homeopathy,* 24 (1931), 1040-43.

28. Julia M. Green, "For the Layman," *Homeopathic Recorder,* 51 (1936), 427-28.

29. Julia M. Green, "For the Laymen," *Homeopathic Recorder,* 52 (1937), 235-36.

30. Green, "For the Laymen," 43-44.

31. Green, "Homeopathy Optimistic," 421-23.

32. Green, "For the Laymen," 326; 282-83.

33. Stuart Close, "The Educational Value of Platforms," *Homeopathic Recorder,* 37 (1922), 560-64.
34. "Editorial," *Homeopathic Recorder,* 52 (1937), 526-27.
35. "Editorial," 527.
36. Eugene Underhill, Jr., "President's Address," *Homeopathic Recorder,* 52 (1937), 388-89. See also Hilary Arksey, "Expert and Lay Participation in the Construction of Medical Knowledge," *Sociology of Health and Illness,* 16 (1994), 448-68.
37. Carl H. Enstam, "Rebuilding Homeopathy," *Journal of the American Institute of Homeopathy,* 33 (1940), 330.
38. Enstam, "Rebuilding Homeopathy," 334.
39. J. W. Waffensmith, "Homeopathic Values in a Changing World," *Journal of the American Institute of Homeopathy,* 37 (1944), 64-65. See also Frederick M. Dearborn (ed.), *American Homeopathy in the World War* (Chicago: American Institute of Homeopathy, 1923).
40. "Pan American Homeopathic Medical Congress, October 25, 1945," *Journal of the American Institute of Homeopathy,* 39 (1946), 96.
41. "Minutes, Annual Meeting of Women's National Homeopathic League," *Journal of the American Institute of Homeopathy,* 61 (1968), 187.
42. Elinore C. Peebles and Edith S. Capon, "Correspondence," *Journal of the American Institute of Homeopathy,* 49 (1956), 91.
43. Elizabeth Stuart Close, "Homeopathic Laymen's League of New York," *Journal of the American Institute of Homeopathy,* 46 (1953), 93.
44. "Report of Delegates' Meeting Layman's Bureau, AIH," *Journal of the American Institute of Homeopathy,* 50 (1957), 285.
45. "News," *Journal of the American Institute of Homeopathy,* 56 (1963), 405; "A Trial Balloon," *Journal of the American Institute of Homeopathy,* 57 (1964), 22.
46. "A New Homeopathic Publication," *Homeopathic Recorder,* 41 (1926), 570-72.
47. Rudolph F. Rabe, "The Outlook of Homeopathy," *The Layman Speaks,* 5 (1952), 7; "Arthur Brooks Green, 49 Years Dedicated to Homeopathy," *The Layman Speaks,* 28 (1974), 241-43.
48. Rudolph F. Rabe, "What Does Homeopathy Have to Offer to the Inquiring Layman?" *The Layman Speaks,* I (1948), 1-7.
49. Arthur Brooks Green, "Layman's Bureau," *The Layman Speaks,* II (1949), 19-20.
50. Rabe, "The Outlook for Homeopathy," 3-8.
51. Edith Capon, "The Problem of Educating Laymen in Homeopathic Philosophy," *The Layman Speaks,* 8 (1955), 150-55.
52. RMD, "Editorial," *The Layman Speaks,* 29 (1976), 195. See also Luther Griffin Jones, "The Law and Homeopathy," *The Layman Speaks,* 29 (1976), 196-97.
53. Alain Naudé, "Editorial," *The Layman Speaks,* 30 (1977), 5-6.
54. Forrest Murphy, "An Interested Look at Homeopathy," *Journal of the American Institute of Homeopathy,* 61 (1968), 40-41.
55. Murphy, "An Interested Look at Homeopathy," 42. The twelve Schüssler cell-salts are Fluoride of Calcium, Phosphate of Calcium, Sulphate of Calcium, Phosphate of Iron, Chloride of Potassium, Phosphate of Potassium, Sulphate of Potassium, Phosphate of Magnesia, Chloride of Sodium, Sulphate of Sodium, and

Silicic Acid. See J. W. Cogswell, *Home Treatment with the Schüssler Remedies* (St. Louis, MO: Luyties Pharmacal Company, n.d.).

56. Murphy, "An Interested Look at Homeopathy," 43.

57. Roger A. Schmidt, "Quo Vadis or Some Consideration on the Past and Future of Homeopathy in the USA," *Journal of the American Institute of Homeopathy,* 61 (1968), 108-109.

58. "Editorial," *Journal of the American Institute of Homeopathy,* 70 (1977), 382-83.

59. "Editorial," 384-85.

60. "Editorial," 194.

Chapter 4

1. William Gutman, "International Institute for Homeopathic Research," *Journal of the American Institute of Homeopathy,* 41 (1948), 93-95.

2. Robert H. Farley, "Homeopathic Research," *Journal of the American Institute of Homeopathy,* 41 (1948), 11-12.

3. C. P. Bryant, "Scientific Knowledge of Vibrations Will Cure and Will Prove the Teachings of Samuel Hahnemann," *Journal of the American Institute of Homeopathy,* 46 (1953), 268-69.

4. "Homeopathy and the Atomic Bomb," *Journal of the American Institute of Homeopathy,* 39 (1946), 19-20.

5. K. C. Hiteshi, "Atomic Bomb and Homeopathy," *Journal of the American Institute of Homeopathy,* 39 (1946), 21-22.

6. William P. Mowry, "The Atomic Energy Principles in the Treatment of the Patient," *Journal of the American Institute of Homeopathy,* 39 (1946), 346-48.

7. Fred B. Morgan, "President's Page," *Journal of the American Institute of Homeopathy,* 40 (1947), 21.

8. A. H. Grimmer, "Homeopathy's Place in Medicine," *Journal of the American Institute of Homeopathy,* 49 (1956), 103.

9. Amaro Azevedo, "Endocrinology—Biochemistry—Nuclear Energy and Homeopathy," *Journal of the American Institute of Homeopathy,* 46 (1953), 334-35, 338.

10. J. D. Vaishnav, "Homeopathy: The Science and the Art," *Homeopathy for Health and Life,* 17 (1968), 79-80.

11. Arthur W. Wase and Jens A. Christensen, "The Significance of Isotopes as New Tools in Homeopathic Research Work," *Journal of the American Institute of Homeopathy,* 48 (1955), 295.

12. Mary I. Senseman, "Homeopathy in the Atomic Age," *Journal of the American Institute of Homeopathy,* 49 (1956), 82-83.

13. Horace E. Reed, "Repetition of the Remedy," *Journal of the American Institute of Homeopathy,* 56 (1963), 200.

14. Roger A. Schmidt, "Some Aspects of Homeopathic Posology in Low Potencies," *Journal of the American Institute of Homeopathy,* 60 (1967), 235.

15. "The Growing Use of NMR for Molecular Research," *Journal of the American Institute of Homeopathy,* 61 (1968), 196; Rudolph B. Smith, Jr., and Garth W. Boericke, "Changes Caused by Succussion on NMR Patterns and Bioassay of

Bradykinin Triacetate (BKTA) Successions and Dilutions," *Journal of the American Institute of Homeopathy,* 61 (1968), 197-212; A. D. Sacks, "Nuclear Magnetic Resonance Spectroscopy of Homeopathic Remedies," *Journal of Holistic Medicine,* 5 (1983), 172-77; J. M. Young, "Nuclear Magnetic Resonance Studies of Succussed Solutions," *Journal of the American Institute of Homeopathy,* 68 (1975), 8-16.

16. A. H. Grimmer, "Our Expanding Homeopathic Philosophy," *Journal of the American Institute of Homeopathy,* 48 (1955), 274.

17. Allen C. Neiswander, "A New Key for an Old Lock," *Journal of the American Institute of Homeopathy,* 47 (1954), 90-91.

18. Christopher Kent Johannes, "Beyond the Avogadro Limit; Homeopathy's Quantum Leap into a New Era of Medicine," *Journal of the American Institute of Homeopathy,* 89 (1996), 151.

19. B. K. Sarkar, "Homeopathy and the Human Organism," *Journal of the American Institute of Homeopathy,* 45 (1952), 182-88.

20. B. K. Sarkar, "The Place of Homeopathy in the Science of Medicine," *Journal of the American Institute of Homeopathy,* 46 (1953), 205-213.

21. Tariq Kuraishy, "Insights into the Homeopathic Philosophy via Eastern Beliefs and Modern Science," *Journal of the American Institute of Homeopathy,* 74 (1981), 13-16.

22. Quoted in Dr. A. V. Subramanian, "Homeopathy and Indian Culture," *The Homeopathy,* 11 (1962), 16, 18-19. See also J. Kishore, "Homeopathy: The Indian Experience," *World Health Forum,* 4 (1983), 105-107; D. Vasant Lad, *Ayuraveda* (Santee Fe, New Mexico: Lotus Press, 1984); D. Vasant Lad, "Ayurvedic Medicine," in Wayne B. Jonas and Jeffrey S. Levin (eds.), *Essentials of Complementary and Alternative Medicine* (Philadelphia: Lippincott Williams and Wilkins, 1999), 200-215.

23. Kuraishy, "Insights into the Homeopathic Philosophy via Eastern Beliefs and Modern Science," 18-19, 25-27. See also P. Bellavite and A. Signorini, *Homeopathy: A Frontier in Medical Science* (Berkeley: North Atlantic Books, 1995).

24. Julian Winston, "Keeping It Alive: Homeopathy Through the First Half of the Century," *Journal of the American Institute of Homeopathy,* 92 (1999), 227.

25. George Vithoulkas, *The Science of Homeopathy* (New York: Grove Press, 1980), xvi.

26. Vithoulkas, *The Science of Homeopathy,* 4, 20, chapter 3.

27. Vithoulkas, *The Science of Homeopathy,* 59, 73-74. See also B. Singer, "Kirlian Photography," in G. Abell and B. Singer (eds.), *Science and the Paranormal* (London: Junction Books, 1981).

28. Vithoulkas, *The Science of Homeopathy,* chapter 5.

29. Vithoulkas, *The Science of Homeopathy,* 97-98, 104.

30. Vithoulkas, *The Science of Homeopathy,* 154-56. See also Tomás Pablo Paschero, *Homeopathy* (Beaconsfield, Bucks UK: Beaconsfield Pub. LTD, 2000), 15-21.

31. Dr. J. Kunzli von Fimelsberg, "Impressions of Homeopathy in the United States," *Journal of the American Institute of Homeopathy,* 75 (1982), 42-43.

32. Kunzli von Fimelsberg, "Impressions of Homeopathy in the United States," 43.

33. George A. Guess, "Letter to Editor," *Journal of the American Institute of Homeopathy,* 75 (1982), 37.

34. Alan Levine, "Letters to the Editor," *Journal of the American Institute of Homeopathy,* 75 (1982), 55-56.

35. David Warkentin and Bill Gray, "The Hahnemann Medical Clinic and Homeopathic Education," *Journal of the American Institute of Homeopathy,* 78 (1985), 34.

36. Henry N. Williams, "Guest Editorial," *Journal of the American Institute of Homeopathy,* 77 (1984), 126.

37. Gustav F. Tufo, "What is Psychotherapy?" *Journal of the American Institute of Homeopathy,* 46 (1953), 369-71. See also William Aron, "Homeopathy, Psychoanalysis and Medical Hypnosis," *The Layman Speaks,* 12 (1959), 411-21.

38. William P. Britsch, Jr., "Editorial," *Journal of the American Institute of Homeopathy,* 41 (1948), 203.

39. A. H. Grimmer, "Homeopathic Psychosomatic Medicine," *Journal of the American Institute of Homeopathy,* 46 (1953), 13-14.

40. Johannes, "Beyond the Avogadro Limit; Homeopathy's Quantum Leap into a New Era of Medicine," 10-13.

41. Bernardo A. Merizalde, "Homeopathy, Alchemy and the Process of Transformation," *Journal of the American Institute of Homeopathy,* 90 (1997), 120-25.

42. Domenick J. Masiello, "Homeopathy: Medicine of the 21st Century," *Journal of the American Institute of Homeopathy,* 91 (1998), 178-80. See also James L. Oschman, *Energy Medicine: The Scientific Basis* (Edinburgh: Churchill Livingston, 2000), 139-46.

43. Joel Shepperd, "The Language of Chaos Theory and Complexity Applied to Homeopathy," *American Journal of Homeopathic Medicine,* 96 (2003), 202-203, 205-206.

44. Joel Shepperd, "Chaos Theory: Implications for Homeopathy," *Journal of the American Institute of Homeopathy,* 87 (1994), 22. See also C. Garner and N. Hock, "Chaos Theory and Homeopathy," *Berlin Journal of Research in Homeopathy,* 1 (1991), 236-42; Prigogine and I. Stengles, *Order Out of Chaos* (New York: Bantam, 1984).

45. Johannes, "Beyond the Avogadro Limit; Homeopathy's Quantum Leap into a New Era of Medicine," 152.

46. Johannes, "Beyond the Avogadro Limit; Homeopathy's Quantum Leap into a New Era of Medicine," 152.

47. Johannes, "Beyond the Avogadro Limit; Homeopathy's Quantum Leap into a New Era of Medicine," 155.

48. Victor M. Margutti, "Homeopathy, Homeotherapeutics and Modern Medicine: A Holistic Approach," *Journal of the American Institute of Homeopathy,* 69 (1976), 200.

49. James Stephenson, "A Review of Investigations into the Action of Substances in Dilutions Greater than 1×10^{-24}," *Journal of the American Institute of Homeopathy,* 71 (1978), 79-94.

50. G. P. Barnard and James H. Stephenson, "Fresh Evidence for a Biophysical Field," *Journal of the American Institute of Homeopathy,* 71 (1978), 67-68.

51. Stephenson, "A Review of Investigations into the Action of Substances in Dilutions Greater than 1×10^{-24}," 96.

52. Matthew Hubbard, "A Mathematical Explanation of the Process of Potentisation," *Journal of the American Institute of Homeopathy,* 71 (1978), 100.

53. Hubbard, "A Mathematical Explanation of the Process of Potentisation," 96-97.

54. Schiff quoted in Timothy Fior, "Book Review," *American Journal of Homeopathic Medicine,* 95 (2002), 37. See also Michel Schiff, *The Memory of Water: Homeopathy and the Battle of Ideas in the New Science* (London: Thorsons, 1995); Robert Park, *Voodoo Science: The Road from Foolishness to Fraud* (New York: Oxford University Press, 2000), 54-58.

55. Timothy Fior, "Book Review," *American Journal of Homeopathic Medicine,* 95 (2002), 40-42; Jacques Benveniste, "Benveniste on the Benveniste Affair," *Nature,* 335 (1988), 759.

56. Daphna Slonim and Kerrin White, "Mainstream Psychiatry and Homeopathy Initiating a Scientific Dialogue," *Journal of the American Institute of Homeopathy,* 75 (1982), 13, 15. See also Jos Kleijnen, Paul Knipschild, and Gerben ter Riet, "Clinical Trials of Homeopathy," *British Medical Journal,* 302 (1991), 316-23.

57. W. B. Jonas, R. L. Anderson, C. C. Crawford, and J. S. Lyons, "A Systematic Review of the Quality of Homeopathic Clinical Trials," *BioMed Central,* 1 (2001), 12. See also H. M. Anthony, "Some Methodological Problems in the Assessment of Complementary Therapy," *Statistics in Medicine,* 6 (1987), 761-71; M. S. Kramer and S. H. Shapiro, "Scientific Challenges in the Application of Randomized Trials," *Journal of the American Medical Association,* 252 (1984), 2739-45.

58. David Taylor Reilly, "Homeopathy and Placebo—A Redundant Hypothesis?" *Journal of the American Institute of Homeopathy,* 83 (1990), 77-79.

59. Jonathan Shore, "Therapeutic Intent, Suggestion, and Placebo," *Journal of the American Institute of Homeopathy,* 83 (1990), 86-88. See also A. Grunbaum, "The Placebo Concept," *Behaviour Research and Therapy,* 19 (1981), 157-67; H. K. Beecher, "The Powerful Placebo," *Journal of the American Medical Association,* 159 (1955), 1602-06; D. O'Keefe, "Is Homeopathy a Placebo Response?" *Lancet,* 329 (1986), 1106-07; P. Götzche, "Trials of Homeopathy," *Lancet,* 341 (1993), 1533.

60. Karl Robinson, "Homeopathy as Phenomenalistic Medicine," *Journal of the American Institute of Homeopathy,* 85 (1992), 14-16.

61. Bill Gray, "Letters to Editor," *Journal of the American Institute of Homeopathy,* 85 (1992), 55.

62. "It Is Higher Science," *Homeopathic Recorder,* 14 (1899), 20.

63. "Alternative Medicine Meets Science," *Journal of the American Medical Association,* 280 (1998), 1618.

64. Quoted in Jennifer Jacobs, "Homeopathic Research: Fact or Fantasy?" *American Journal of Homeopathic Medicine,* 95 (2002), 26. See also D. Eisenberg, R. C. Kessler, and C. Foster, "Unconventional Medicine in the United States," *New England Journal of Medicine,* 328 (1993), 246-52.

65. Jennifer Jacobs, "Future Directions in Homeopathic Research," *Journal of the American Institute of Homeopathy,* 87 (1994), 156.

66. Jennifer Jacobs, "President's Message: Homeopathic Research With Heart," *Journal of the American Institute of Homeopathy,* 94 (2001), 88. 90-91; Wayne B. Jonas and Jennifer Jacobs, *Healing with Homeopathy: The Complete Guide* (New York: Warner Books, 1996), 84-94.

67. Jacobs, "Homeopathic Research: Fact or Fantasy?" 30.

68. Jennifer Jacobs and Richard Moskowitz, "Homeopathy," in Marc S. Micozzi (ed.), *Fundamentals of Complementary and Alternative Medicine* (New York and London: Churchill Livingstone, 1996), 75.

69. Jacobs and Moskowitz, "Homeopathy," 76.

70. Richard Pitcairn, "Homeopathy: Antidote to a Materialistic Age," *Journal of the American Institute of Homeopathy,* 93 (2000), 7-9, 20-21; Julian Winston, *The Faces of Homeopathy: An Illustrated History of the First 200 Years* (Tawa, New Zealand: Great Auk Publishers, 1999), 447-53.

71. Randall Neustaedter, "Perspectives on Classical Homeopathy," *Journal of the American Institute of Homeopathy,* 80 (1987), 66-67. See also Harris L. Coulter, *The Controlled Clinical Trial: An Analysis* (Washington, D.C.: Center for Empirical Medicine, 1991).

72. Andrew Weil, *Health and Healing* (Boston: Houghton Mifflin Company, 1983), 37.

Chapter 5

1. Allan D. Sutherland, "Allopathy," *Journal of the American Institute of Homeopathy,* 49 (1956), 281.

2. Henry W. Eisfelder, "President's Message," *Journal of the American Institute for Homeopathy,* 49 (1956), 117, 153.

3. "A Warning," *Journal of the American Institute of Homeopathy,* 50 (1957), 117.

4. Donald G. Gladish, "The President's Message," *Journal of the American Institute of Homeopathy,* 51 (1958), 108.

5. Wyrth Post Baker, "The Place of Homeopathy in American Medicine," *Journal of the American Institute of Homeopathy,* 50 (1957), 296-98.

6. Henry W. Eisfelder, "Today's Trend in Homeopathy," *Journal of the American Institute of Homeopathy,* 43 (1950), 221-22.

7. Paul S. Schantz, "What Does Homeopathy Need?" *Journal of the American Institute of Homeopathy,* 48 (1955), 78.

8. Mahboob Alam Qureshi, "Homeopathy All Over the World," *The Layman Speaks,* 18 (1965), 48.

9. A. H. Grimmer, "President's Message," *Journal of the American Institute of Homeopathy,* 47 (1954), 182-83.

10. A. C. N., "The Forward Look," *Journal of the American Institute of Homeopathy,* 48 (1955), 89-90.

11. "A Time for Decision," *Journal of the American Institute of Homeopathy,* 48 (1955), 314.

12. "Editorial," *Journal of the American Institute of Homeopathy,* 50 (1957), 85.

13. "The Homeopathic Recorder," *Journal of the American Institute of Homeopathy,* 57 (1964), 169. See also Julian Winston, *The Faces of Homeopathy: An Illustrated History of the First 200 Years* (Tawa, New Zealand: Great Awk Publishers, 1999), 311-13.

14. "Editorial," *Journal of the American Institute of Homeopathy,* 50 (1957), 313.

15. "The Future," *Journal of the American Institute of Homeopathy,* 56 (1963), 278.

16. W. W. Young, "Some Thoughts About the Future," *Journal of the American Institute of Homeopathy,* 56 (1963), 283-84.

17. W. W. Young, "J' Accuse," *Journal of the American Institute of Homeopathy,* 64 (1971), 130-31.

18. W. W. Young, "Co-Existence," *Journal of the American Institute of Homeopathy,* 60 (1967), 140-42.

19. W. W. Young, "The Perpetuation and Propagation Program," *Journal of the American Institute of Homeopathy,* 60 (1967), 200-201.

20. Young, "The Perpetuation and Propagation Program," 202, 204-207.

21. Frederic Schmidt, "President's Address," *Journal of the American Institute of Homeopathy,* 72 (1979), 197-98.

22. Frederic W. Schmidt, "Thoughts from Your President," *Journal of the American Institute of Homeopathy,* 73 (1980), 5-6.

23. Jack Cooper, "Thoughts from the President," *Journal of the American Institute of Homeopathy,* 74 (1981), 5.

24. Hela Michot-Dietrich, "Letter to Editor," *Journal of the American Institute of Homeopathy,* 78 (1985), 53.

25. Julian Winston, "Letter to the Editor," *Journal of the American Institute of Homeopathy,* 78 (1985), 139.

26. Franklin McCoy, "Letter to the Editor," *Journal of the American Institute of Homeopathy,* 81 (1988), 62-63.

27. Domenick John Masiello, "Letter to the Editor," *Journal of the American Institute of Homeopathy,* 82 (1989), 87-88.

28. Edward Chapman, "A Message from the President," *Journal of the American Institute of Homeopathy,* 84 (1991), 89-90.

29. Guy Hoagland, "Homeotherapeutics: A New Perspective," *Journal of the American Institute of Homeopathy,* 85 (1992), 12-13.

30. Guy Hoagland, "Opinion: Homeopathy—Medicine or Religion?" *Journal of the American Institute of Homeopathy,* 86 (1993), 194-95.

31. Hoagland, "Opinion: Homeopathy—Medicine or Religion?" 195.

32. Hoagland, "Opinion: Homeopathy—Medicine or Religion?" 195-96.

33. Edward Chapman, "Message from the President," *Journal of the American Institute of Homeopathy,* 87 (1994), 63-64.

34. Randall Neustaedter, "Opinion," *Journal of the American Institute of Homeopathy,* 87 (19), 66-67.

35. Karl Robinson, "Letter to the Editor," *Journal of the American Institute of Homeopathy,* 87 (1994), 190.

36. Richard Moskowitz, "Who Needs the AIH? A Brief Pep Talk," *Journal of the American Institute of Homeopathy,* 87 (1994), 193, 196.

37. Richard Moskowitz, "Ethics in Homeopathic Practice," *Journal of the American Institute of Homeopathy,* 86 (1993), 238.

38. Sandra M. Chase, "President's Message," *Journal of the American Institute of Homeopathy,* 91 (1998), 213. See also Isabell Biddle, "The Inter-Relationship Between Osteopathy and Homeopathy," *The Layman Speaks,* 20 (1967), 325-28.

39. Edward Chapman, "President's Letter," *Journal of the American Institute of Homeopathy,* 88 (1995), 165-66.

40. Edward Chapman, "Homeopathy—Moving Towards the Mainstream in a Changing Health Care System," *Journal of the American Institute of Homeopathy,* 88 (1995), 174.

41. Suzanne White Junod, "An Alternative Perspective; Homeopathic Drugs, Royal Copeland, and Federal Drug Regulation," *Food and Drug Law Journal,* 55 (2000), 168-69.

42. "Editorial," 385-86.

43. Henry N. Williams, "Guest Editorial," *Journal of the American Institute of Homeopathy,* 78 (1985), 49.

44. J. P. Borneman, "The Regulation of Homeopathy: A Perspective," *Journal of the American Institute of Homeopathy,* 80 (1987), 32-35. See also E. Ernst, "Bitter Pills of Nature: Safety Issues in Complementary Medicine," *Pain,* 60 (1995), 237-38.

45. "President's Message," *Journal of the American Institute of Homeopathy,* 88 (1995), 5-6.

46. Chapman, "Homeopathy—Moving Towards the Mainstream in a Changing Health Care System," 173.

47. Edward Chapman, "President's Message," *Journal of the American Institute of Homeopathy,* 89 (1996), 6-7.

48. Edward Chapman, "President's Message," *Journal of the American Institute of Homeopathy,* 90 (1997), 5-6.

49. Chapman, "President's Message," 6.

50. Edward Chapman, "A President's Parting Words: The Community of Homeopathy," *Journal of the American Institute of Homeopathy,* 90 (1997), 117-18.

51. Sandra M. Chase, "President's Message," *Journal of the American Institute of Homeopathy,* 91 (1998), 305.

52. Jennifer Jacobs, "President's Message: Homeopathic Research with Heart," *Journal of the American Institute of Homeopathy,* 94 (2001), 88.

53. Jennifer Jacobs, "Bringing Homeopathy to More People," *American Journal of Homeopathic Medicine,* 95 (2002), 4.

54. Iris R. Bell, "Evidence-Based Homeopathy: Empirical Questions and Methodological Considerations for Homeopathic Clinical Research," *American Journal of Homeopathic Medicine,* 96 (2003), 17-31.

55. Jennifer Jacobs, "Reflections after 25 Years of Homeopathic Practice," *American Journal of Homeopathic Medicine,* 96 (2003), 6-7.

56. Jennifer Jacobs, "President's Report—WCCAM to Issue Interim Report," *Journal of the American Institute of Homeopathy,* 94 (2001), 157.

57. Jared L. Zeff, "Letters to Editor," *Journal of the American Institute of Homeopathy,* 78 (1985), 51.

58. Durr Elmore, "Naturopathy and Homeopathy," *Journal of the American Institute of Homeopathy,* 85 (1992), 60-63. See also G. Cody, "History of Naturopathic Medicine,' in Joseph E. Pizzorno and Michael T. Murray, *A Textbook of Natural Medicine* (Seattle, Washington: John Bastyr College Publications, 1985).

59. Because of inconsistencies in state laws, some individuals who attended chiropractic colleges discovered they could use the title of naturopath without ever having set foot in a naturopathic school. Indeed, there were instances of individuals presenting themselves as naturopathic physicians and using the initials ND without having received a diploma from any of the established schools. The only way one could make sure that the person with the ND was real was to call the American Association of Naturopathic Physicians in Seattle to verify that the person was licensed.

60. Elmore, "Naturopathy and Homeopathy," 60-63.

61. Edward H. Chapman, "AIH Position Paper on Naturopathic Practice," *Journal of the American Institute of Homeopathy,* 86 (1993), 138.

62. Greg Bedayn, "Letter to the Editor," *Journal of the American Institute of Homeopathy,* 90 (1997), 69.

63. Today, there are forty-four institutions teaching homeopathy spread across sixteen states, Ontario, and British Columbia.

64. Joel Kreisberg, "Trends in Homeopathic Education: A Survey of Homeopathic Schools in North America 1998," *Journal of the American Institute of Homeopathy,* 93 (2000), 75-84.

65. Joyce Frye, "Put the Moose on the Table," *American Journal of Homeopathic Medicine,* 96 (2003), 185-86.

Chapter 6

1. George Guess, "Editorial Preface," *American Journal of Homeopathic Medicine,* 95 (2002), 58.

2. Jennifer Jacobs, "Lets Agree to Disagree—With Respect," *American Journal of Homeopathic Medicine,* 95 (2002), 60.

3. Richard Moskowitz, "An Issue That Won't Go Away," *American Journal of Homeopathic Medicine,* 97 (2004), 27-28.

4. Roger Morrison, Jonathan Shore, Nancy Herrick, Rajan Sankaran, Stephen King, Ted Chapman, Mitchell Fleisher, Ed Kondrot, David Riley, Duncan Soule, Declan Hammond, Jeff Baker, Deborah Gordon, Melissa Fairbanks, Corrie Hiwat, Harry van der Zee, Andrew Bonner, Rebecca Reese, Richard Moskowitz, Eric Sommerman, Deborah Collins, "Against Divisiveness," *Homeopathy Today,* 21 (2001), 21-22. See also Julian Winston, "Editorial," *Homeopathy Today,* 20 (2000), 21-22; André Saine, "Homeopathy vs. Speculative Medicine: A Call to Action," *Simillimum,* 14 (2001), 34-54.

5. André Saine, "Drawing a Line in the Sand: Homeopathy or Not Homeopathy?" *American Journal of Homeopathic Medicine,* 95 (2002), 72.

6. Quoted in Saine, "Drawing a Line in the Sand: Homeopathy or Not Homeopathy?" 72.

7. Saine, "Drawing a Line in the Sand: Homeopathy or Not Homeopathy?" 74.
8. Saine, "Drawing a Line in the Sand: Homeopathy or Not Homeopathy?" 76, 82.
9. Saine, "Drawing a Line in the Sand: Homeopathy or Not Homeopathy?" 84.
10. Saine, "Drawing a Line in the Sand: Homeopathy or Not Homeopathy?" 84.
11. Quoted in André Saine, "Fads, Trends, and Dogma Undermining the Quality of the Practice of Homeopathy in America," *Journal of the American Institute of Homeopathy,* 87 (1994), 200.
12. Saine, "Fads, Trends, and Dogma Undermining the Quality of the Practice of Homeopathy in America," 203-205.
13. Morrison et al., "Against Divisiveness," 21-22.
14. Roger Morrison, "Forum: Controversy in Homeopathy," *American Journal of Homeopathic Medicine,* 95 (2002), 65-66.
15. Morrison, "Forum: Controversy in Homeopathy," 88, 90.
16. Klaus Habich, Curt Kosters, and Jochen Rohwer, "Magic or Science," *American Journal of Homeopathic Medicine,* 96 (2003), 82.
17. Habich, Kosters, and Rohwer, "Magic or Science," 83.
18. Habich, Kosters, and Rohwer, "Magic or Science," 84.
19. Habich, Kosters, and Rohwer, "Magic or Science," 86-87.
20. Habich, Kosters, and Rohwer, "Magic or Science," 87, 89.
21. Habich, Kosters, and Rohwer, "Magic or Science," 88.
22. Richard Moskowitz, "Innovation and Fundamentalism in Homeopathy," *American Journal of Homeopathic Medicine,* 95 (2002), 92-93.
23. J. H. Renner, "Correspondence," *Journal of the American Institute of Homeopathy,* 60 (1967), 247. For example of the use by the laity, see T. Douglas Ross, "Spotting the Remedy," *The Layman Speaks,* 22 (1969), 14-17.
24. Moskowitz, "Innovation and Fundamentalism in Homeopathy," 94, 103.
25. Moskowitz, "Innovation and Fundamentalism in Homeopathy," 103.
26. Moskowitz, "Innovation and Fundamentalism in Homeopathy," 107.
27. Moskowitz, "An Issue That Won't Go Away," 31-32.
28. Moskowitz, "An Issue That Won't Go Away," 35, 44, 46.
29. Julian Winston, "Comments on the Controversy," *American Journal of Homeopathic Medicine,* 95 (2002), 187.

Bibliography

Journals

American Journal of Health
American Homeopathic Observer
American Homeopathic Review
American Journal of Homeopathic Medicine
Behaviour Research and Therapy
Berlin Journal of Research in Homeopathy
BioMed Central
British Homeopathic Journal
British Medical Journal
Bulletin of the History of Medicine
Church History
Food and Drug Law Journal
Hahnemannian Monthly
Homeopathic Heartbeat
Homeopathic Links
Homeopathic Recorder
Homeopathic Recorder
Homeopathic Survey
Homeopathy
Homeopathy Today
Homeopathy for Health and Life
Homeotherapy
Journal of Holistic Medicine
Journal of the American Institute of Homeopathy
Journal of the American Medical Association
Journal of the History of Medicine
Lancet
Layman Speaks
Layman's Bulletin
Laymen's Weekly
Medical Advance
New England Journal of Medicine
Pacific Coast Journal of Homeopathy
Pain

Pennsylvania Magazine of History and Biography
Report, U.S. Bureau of Education
Simillimum
Sociology of Health and Illness
Statistics in Medicine
World Health Forum

Books

Abrahams, Albert. *New Concepts in Diagnosis and Treatment.* San Francisco: Philopolis Press, 1916.
Allen, Henry C. *The Materia Medica of the Nosodes with Provings of the X-ray.* Philadelphia: Boericke and Tafel, 1910.
Barnard, Julian. *Bach Flower Remedies: Form and Function.* Massachusetts: Lindisfarne Books, 2004.
Bellavite, P., and A. Signorini. *Homeopathy: A Frontier in Medical Science.* Berkeley: North Atlantic Books, 1995.
Boericke, William, and A. Willis Dewey. *The Twelve Tissue Remedies of Schüssler.* Philadelphia: Boericke and Tafel, 1893.
Boyd, W. E. *Research on the Low Potencies of Homeopathy.* London: William Heinemann, 1936.
Brown, E. Richard. *Rockefeller Medicine Men: Medicine and Capitalism in America.* Berkeley: University of California Press, 1979.
Burrow, James Gordon. *AMA: Voice of American Medicine.* Baltimore: Johns Hopkins Press, 1963.
Burrow, James Gordon. *Organized Medicine in the Progressive Era: The Move Toward Monopoly.* Baltimore: Johns Hopkins University Press, 1977.
Bynum, W. F., and Roy Porter (eds.). *Medical Fringe and Medical Orthodoxy, 1750-1850.* London: Croom Helm, 1987.
Campbell, Anthony. *The Two Faces of Homeopathy.* London: R. Hale, 1984.
Chopra, Deepak. *Perfect Health: The Complete Mind-Body Guide.* Harmony: Crown, 1990.
Cogswell, J. W. *Home Treatment with the Schüssler Remedies.* St. Louis, Missouri: Luyties Pharmacal Company, n.d.
Cook, Trevor M. *Homeopathic Medicine Today.* New Canaan, Connecticut: Keats Publishing Inc., 1989.
Cooter, Roger, and John Pictstone (Eds.). *Medicine in the Twentieth Century.* Australia: Harwood Academic Publishers, 2000.
Cordasco, Franscesco (Ed.). *Homeopathy in the United States: A Bibliography of Homeopathic Medical Imprints, 1825-1925.* Fairview, N. J.: Junius-Vaughn Press, 1991.
Coulter, Harris L. *Divided Legacy: A History of the Schism in Medical Thought. Vol. III. Science and Ethics in American Medicine, 1800-1914.* Washington, D.C.: Wehawken Book Company, 1977.

Coulter, Harris L. *The Controlled Clinical Trial: An Analysis.* Washington, D.C.: Center for Empirical Medicine, 1991.
Dearborn, Frederick M. *American Homeopathy in the World War.* Chicago: American Institute of Homeopathy, 1923.
DeCharms, Richard. *Hahnemann and Swedenborg: Or the Affinities Between the Fundamental Principles of Homeopathia and the Doctrines of the New Church.* Philadelphia: New Jerusalem Printers, 1850.
Dinges, Martin (Ed.). *Patients in the History of Homeopathy.* Sheffield: European Association for the History of Medicine and Health Publications, 2002.
Duffy, John. *The Healers: A History of American Medicine.* Urbana: University of Illinois Press, 1976.
Dunham, Carroll. *Homeopathy, the Science of Therapeutics: A Collection of Papers Elucidating and Illustrating the Principles of Homeopathy.* Calcutta: Haren and Brother, 1973.
Fincke, Bernhardt. *On High Potencies and Homeopathics.* Philadelphia: A. J. Tafel, 1865.
Fishbein, Morris. *Medical Follies.* New York: Boni and Liveright, 1932.
Flexner, Abraham. *Medical Education in the United States and Canada; A Report to the Carnegie Foundation for the Advancement of Teaching.* New York: Carnegie Foundation for the Advancement of Teaching, 1910.
Fuller, Robert C. *Alternative Medicine and American Religious Life.* New York: Oxford University Press, 1989.
Gevitz, Norman (Ed.). *Other Healers: Unorthodox Medicine in America.* Baltimore: Johns Hopkins University Press, 1988.
Hall, A. Wilford. *The Problem of Human Life.* New York: Hall and Company, 1877.
Haller, Jr., John S. *A Profile in Alternative Medicine: The Eclectic Medical College of Cincinnati, 1845-1942.* Kent, Ohio: Kent State University Press, 1999.
Haller, Jr., John S. *The History of American Homeopathy: The Academic Years, 1820-1936.* Binghamton, New York: Haworth Press Inc., 2005.
Haller, Jr., John S. *The People's Doctors: Samuel Thomson and the American Botanical Movement, 1790-1860.* Carbondale: Southern Illinois University Press, 2000.
Harvey, C. G., and A. Cochrane. *The Encyclopedia of Flower Remedies.* London: Thorson's, 1995.
Hering, Constantine. *The Twelve Tissue Remedies and Their Use in the Trituration of Dr. Schüssler.* New York: Boericke and Tafel, 1874.
Hughes, Richard. *Manual of Pharmacodynamics.* 6th ed.; London: Leath and Ross, 1983.
Johnston, Robert D. (Ed.). *The Politics of Healing.* New York: Routledge, 2004.
Jonas, Wayne B., and Jeffrey S. Levin (Eds.). *Essentials of Complementary and Alternative Medicine.* Philadelphia: Lippincott Williams and Wilkins, 1999.
Jonas, Wayne B., and Jennifer Jacobs. *Healing with Homeopathy: The Complete Guide.* New York: Warner Books, 1996.
Judah, J. Stillson. *The History and Philosophy of the Metaphysical Movements in America.* Philadelphia: Westminster Press, 1967.

Jütte, Robert, Guenter B. Risse, and John Woodward (Eds.). *Culture, Knowledge, and Healing: Historical Perspectives of Homeopathic Medicine in Europe and North America.* Sheffield: EAHMA, 1998.

Jütte, Robert, Motzi Eklöf, and Marie C. Nelson (Eds.). *Historical Aspects of Unconventional Medicine.* Sheffield: EAHMH, 2001.

Kaufman, Martin. *Homeopathy in America: The Rise and Fall of a Medical Heresy.* Baltimore: Johns Hopkins University Press, 1971.

Kayne, Steven B. *Complementary Therapies for Pharmacists.* London: Pharmaceutical Press, 2002.

Kent, James Tyler. *The Art and Science of Homeopathic Medicine.* Mineola, New York: Dover Publications, Inc., 2002.

Kent, James Tyler. *Lectures on Homeopathic Materia Medica.* New Delhi: Jain Publishing Company, 1980.

Kent, James Tyler. *Repertory of the Homeopathic Materia Medica.* New Delhi: World Homeopathic Links, 1982.

Kirchfeld, Friedhelm, and Wade Boyle. *Nature Doctors: Pioneers in Naturopathic Medicine.* Portland, Oregon: Medicina Biologica, 1994.

Kirschmann, Ann Taylor. *A Vital Force: Women in American Homeopathy.* New Brunswick, New Jersey: Rutgers University Press, 2004.

Kruger, Helen. *Other Healers, Other Cures: A Guide to Alternative Medicine.* Indianapolis: Bobbs-Merrill, 1974.

Lad, Vasant. *Ayurveda: The Science of Self-Healing: A Practical Guide.* Santee Fe, NM: Lotus Press, 1984.

Larsen, Robin (Ed.). *Emanuel Swedenborg: A Continuing Vision.* New York: Swedenborg Foundation, 1988.

Ludmerer, Kenneth M. *Learning to Heal: The Development of American Medical Education.* New York: Basic Books, 1985.

Mansfield, P. *Flower Remedies.* London: Optima, 1995.

Marks, Harry M. *The Progress of Experiment: Science and Therapeutic Reform in the United States, 1900-1990.* Cambridge: Cambridge University Press, 1997.

Mattson, Phyllis H. *Holistic Health in Perspective.* Palo Alto, California: Mayfield, 1982.

McGavack, Thomas Hodge. *The Homeopathic Principle in Therapeutics.* Philadelphia: Boericke and Tafel, 1932.

Micozzi, Marc S. (Ed.). *Fundamentals of Complementary and Alternative Medicine.* New York and London: Churchill Livingstone, 1996.

Moore, R. Laurence. *In Search of White Crows: Spiritualism, Parapsychology, and American Culture.* New York: Oxford University Press, 1977.

National College of Naturopathic Medicine. *Catalog.* Portland, Oregon, n.d.

Nicholls, Phillip A. *Homeopathy and the Medical Profession.* London: Croom Helm, 1988.

O'Connor, B. B. *Healing Traditions, Alternative Medicines and the Health Professions.* Philadelphia: University of Pennsylvania Press, 1995.

Office of Alternative Medicine. *Alternative Medicine: Expanding Medical Horizons.* Bethesda, Maryland: Office of Alternative Medicine, National Institute of Health, 1992.

Oschman, James L. *Energy Medicine: The Scientific Basis.* Edinburgh: Churchill Livingston, 2000.
Park, Robert. *Voodoo Science: The Road from Foolishness to Fraud.* New York: Oxford University Press, 2000.
Paschero, Tomás Pablo. *Homeopathy.* Beaconsfield, Bucks, U.K: Beaconsfield Pub. Ltd, 2000.
Prigogine, I., and I. Stengles. *Order Out of Chaos.* New York: Bantam, 1984.
Roberts, Herbert A. *The Principles and Art of Cure by Homeopathy.* Halsworthy, England: Health Science Press, 1942.
Robins, Natalie. *Copeland's Cure: Homeopathy and the War Between Conventional and Alternative Medicine.* New York: Alfred A. Knopf, 2005.
Rogers, Naomi. *An Alternative Path: The Making and Remaking of Hahnemann Medical College and Hospital of Philadelphia.* New Brunswick: Rutgers University Press, 1998.
Rohland, Robert. *Od, or Odo-Magnetic, Force: An Explanation of Its Influence on Homeopathic Medicines, From the Odic Point of View.* New York: n.p., 1871.
Rothstein, William G. *American Medical Schools and the Practice of Medicine.* New York: Oxford University Press, 1987.
Salmon, J. Warren (Ed.). *Alternative Medicines: Popular and Policy Perspectives.* New York: Tavistock, 1984.
Scheffer, Mechthild. *Bach Flower Therapy: Theory and Practice.* Rochester, Vermont: Healing Arts Press, 1988.
Schiff, Michel. *The Memory of Water: Homeopathy and the Battle of Ideas in the New Sciences.* London: Thorsons, 1995.
Shapiro, Jeffrey G. *The Flower Remedy Book.* Berkeley: North Atlantic Books, 1999.
Stalker, D., and C. Clymour (Eds.). *Examining Holistic Medicine.* Buffalo: Prometheus, 1985.
Starr, Paul. *The Social Transformation of American Medicine.* New York: Basic Books, 1982.
Swan, Samuel. *Catalogue of Morbific Products, Nosodes, and Other Remedies, in High Potencies.* New York: Pusey and Company, 1886.
Swank, Scott Trego. *The Unfettered Conscience, A Study of Sectarianism, Spiritualism and Social Reform in the New Jerusalem Church.* PhD Dissertation, University of Pennsylvania, 1970.
Ullman, Dana. *Discovering Homeopathy: Your Introduction to the Science and Art of Homeopathic Medicine.* Berkeley, California: North Atlantic Books, 1991.
Verspoor, Rudi, and Decker, Steven. *Homeopathy Re-Examined—Beyond the Classical Paradigm.* Ontario, Canada: Hahnemann Center for Heilkunst, 1999.
Vithoulkas, George. *The Science of Homeopathy.* New York: Grove Press, 1980.
Weil, Andrew. *Health and Healing.* Boston: Houghton Mifflin Company, 1983.
Weiner, Michael. *The Complete Book of Homeopathy.* Garden City Park, New York: Avry Publishing Group, Inc., 1989.
Whorton, James C. *Nature Cures: The History of Alternative Medicine in America.* New York: Oxford University Press, 2002.

Wilkinson, Clement John. *John James Garth Wilkinson. A Memoir of His Life with a Selection of His Letters.* London: Kegan Paul Trench Trubner, 1911.

Winston, Julian. *The Faces of Homeopathy: An Illustrated History of the First 200 Years.* Tawa, New Zealand: Great Auk Publishers, 1999.

Wood, Matthew. *The Magical Staff: The Vitalist Tradition in Western Medicine.* Berkeley: North Atlantic, 1992.

Index

About the Author

John S. Haller Jr., PhD, is an emeritus professor of history and medical humanities at Southern Illinois University Carbondale. He has written more than a dozen books on subjects ranging from race to sexuality and the history of medicine. His most recent books include *Swedenborg, Mesmer, and the Mind/Body Connection and The History of New Thought: From Mind Cure to Positive Thinking and the Prosperity Gospel*. He is former editor of *Caduceus: A Humanities Journal for Medicine and the Health Sciences* and, until his retirement in 2008, served for eighteen years as vice president for academic affairs for Southern Illinois University.

CPSIA information can be obtained at www.ICGtesting.com
Printed in the USA
BVOW070837300113

311938BV00002B/5/P